Lithium for Bipolar Disorder

A Guide for Patients

Lithium for Bipolar Disorder

A Guide for Patients

Bipolar Information Series

Dr Nick Stafford

A comprehensive guide to lithium, the evidence for its use in bipolar disorder, its side effects and more

My Mind Books

© 2011

This edition first published 2011 by My Mind Books
My Mind Books Ltd, Four Oaks, UK
Companies House registered private limited company 07769953

ISBN 978-1-908445-00-1
Copyright © 2011 Nick Stafford

The right of Nick Stafford to be identified as the author of this work has been asserted with the Copyright, Design and Patents Act of 1988.

A CIP catalogue record for this book is available from the British Library.

Printed and bound by Lulupress

This book is intended for reference only. It is not a substitute for any medical advice you receive from your medical professionals. You should not alter your medication in any way, or the dose of any of your medication without first consulting your doctor. Mention of products, companies and organisations and the use of images do not employ endorsement of the publisher or imply that these endorse this book. All addresses, websites and telephone numbers in this book were correct at the time of going to press.

My Mind Books Ltd specialises in mental health and wellbeing.

Visit www.mymindbooks.com to read more about our books.

Dedication
To my patients

As we advance in life it becomes more and more difficult,

but in fighting the difficulties

the inmost strength of the heart is developed.

Vincent Van Gogh

Disclaimer

This book is intended for reference only.

It is not a substitute for any medical advice you receive from your medical professionals. You should not alter your medication in any way, or the dose of any of your medication without first consulting your doctor.

Details of the licensing of drugs in this volume and series relate mainly to the UK, unless otherwise stated. In other countries licences for drugs may vary according to the relevant medicines licensing authority for that country.

Acknowledgments

I am eternally grateful to my wife, Toni, and my children who have been patient and supportive while I have written this, my first book. Toni has continued to encourage me in the importance of this volume and also other books that are in preparation for the bipolar information series. She has constantly reminded me of the need to write from my own, and my family's, experiences, and how this has shaped the way we see the needs of other people with the illness.

My parents have remained the immovable cornerstone throughout, with this project, as well with the original idea and series concept. My brother, Chris, as principal editor, has played a key role in the design and house style of My Mind Books and in making the language of the series more understandable to a non-medical audience.

Thank you also to Clare Dolman, chair of Bipolar UK (formerly MDF the Bipolar Organisation) and also to Dr Nicola Rowe, Trustee to the charity for their support and advice.

Thank you to Professor Stephen Bazire, Chief Pharmacist, Norfolk and Waveney Mental Health NHS Foundation Trust, for reviewing the text, for his advice on pharmaceutical technical details and improving the readability of the many complex term used in the book.

I am grateful to Dr Francesc Colom, Head of the Psychoeducation and Psychological Treatments Area at the Barcelona Disorders Programme Clinic, for writing the forward. His renowned work in the psychoeducation of people with bipolar disorder, and how this is reshaping the way we, as clinicians, treat patients throughout the world, has inspired me in both my professional and personal life.

Declaration of interest

The author is in full time employment as a practicing consultant psychiatrist at Leicestershire Partnership NHS Trust, a mental health trust of the National Health Service in the UK. He currently holds no position within a committee that has influence in the prescribing of medication locally, regionally or nationally. He has previously been employed as clinical director in his trust.

He is involved as principal investigator in a number of portfolio research studies in mood disorders and schizophrenia, some of these funded by pharmaceutical companies.

He accepts funding for educational and service development projects from a number of companies in the pharmaceutical industry. These companies have included Sanofi Aventis, Otsuka, Bristol Myers Squibb, AstraZeneca, Eli Lilly, Lundbeck, Pfizer, Servier Laboratories and GW Pharma.

Neither he nor members of his immediate family hold any shares in any pharmaceutical company.

He writes a regular feature, Doctor's Orders, for Mental Health Today, a professionals' magazine published by Pavilion. He also writes for other magazines and newspapers.

He is a Board member of Bipolar UK (formerly MDF the Bipolar Organisation), a UK based charity supporting and providing services to those affected by bipolar disorder. For almost 30 years it has remained the leading and sole UK charity specialising in providing services for those with bipolar disorder in the UK. He accepts no payment for this role.

Contents

Preface

Bipolar Information Series

Guides for patients

This book is a comprehensive guide to how lithium is used to treat bipolar disorder. It is one of a developing range of books in the "A Guide for Patients, The Bipolar Information Series", from My Mind Books.

Here you will find a detailed description of lithium and the evidence for its use in bipolar disorder. This book assumes that you want to know more than your doctors have told you, or have the time to tell you. It contains more detail about side effects than the medication box patient information leaflet .

Written for most readers to understand, this book does not require a medical degree to understand it. If technical words are used, they are explained. The information is written by Dr Nick Stafford, a consultant psychiatrist. He has a clinical and research interest in bipolar disorder, practices psychiatry in the United Kingdom and has 20 years experience in the field of medicine. He is Vice Chair of Bipolar UK (formerly MDF the Bipolar Organisation), the leading national UK bipolar disorder charity.

There is good evidence that quality information and psychoeducation for those with bipolar disorder is proven to improve the overall wellbeing of people with the disorder and also help those involved in their care.

Psychoeducation is learning in detail aspects and details of your illness so that you have a greater understanding of it, are able to manage it better and take better control of your life. This is done with professionals in the form of a course taken over many weeks and is becoming increasingly available around the world.

The aim of this, and other books in the series is to give a detailed account on very specific areas of bipolar disorder. These volumes will be constantly updated and new volumes added.

Patient Guides in the Bipolar Information Series are all available online through Amazon, Lulu and other retail outlets. In time you will be able to purchase them as print versions in other languages and as audio books or download them for use on various eBook readers.

Forward

Lithium, the Salt of the Earth

Dr Francesc Colom

Francesc Colom PsyD, PhD, MSc
Head of Psychoeducation and Psychological Treatments Area
Barcelona Bipolar Disorders Program
IDIBAPS-CIBERSAM

In the beginning there was lithium. A straightforward compound. Not even a compound. A natural salt.

I do not want to talk in depth about the extraordinary oddity of lithium and the magic of the discovery of its mood-stabilising properties made by Dr. John Cade in 1949. Just let me say that this finding, potentially crucial for a good 4% of the world's total population, was made in an abandoned kitchen in an old mental hospital. That was the only resource that the enthusiastic Dr Cade could get when he asked his hospital manager for a lab. And this is the key problem with psychiatry, all over the world. Psychiatry departments are always and everywhere assigned the remotest rooms in the hospital, the windowless offices and the smallest labs.

Why is it so? Are psychiatrists, on average, less intelligent than other medical doctors? Less assertive, so they can not defend their rights and positions? Less politically-skilled to deal with hospital managers? Probably not.

So, why do they get the worst hospital and university facilities? Because psychiatry has been, and in some places still remains, something to hide. It is a stigmatised discipline dealing with stigmatised illnesses.

The daily battle against stigma is psychiatry's major duty. It is, perhaps, the last border to cross in order to reach a full status amongst our colleagues in other areas of medicine. But it is also an unmet need to allow our patients actually have equal rights than other people affected, say, by a neurological or a cardiological condition.

The stigma associated with psychiatric disorders has its roots in the rich soil of ignorance and prejudice and often gets the nutrients it needs from fear. Hence, knowledge dissemination is the only efficacious way of dealing with stigma.

Humankind fears the unknown. Perhaps it is adaptive from an evolutionary perspective. Running from the unknown may keep mankind alive. But, from this same evolutionary perspective, humankind tends to try to understand what is partially known. Running towards knowledge keeps mankind human.

Let's help psychiatric disorders cross this border, so people will move from fearing them to try to understand them and, finally accept them. This is not a minor issue if we consider that up to 4 out of every ten people suffer from some mental disorder if we include soft and milder forms.

This is why I firmly believe that informing the general population is a powerful and underused tool. This is why I devoted my entire professional career to educating people suffering from bipolar disorder on how to accept its condition, live with it, cope with it. Keep it under control.

But let's go back to the beginning. In the beginning there was lithium. To date, lithium is still considered the gold-standard in the maintenance treatment of bipolar disorder. Some colleagues dismiss lithium as an old drug. This is true: lithium is 62 today. So what? Birthday greetings, bottle of wine. This is, by far, an advantage rather than a disadvantage as professionals all over the world benefit from the long experience of using it.

This is the case, for instance, with lithium and pregnancy. It is true that lithium is not a teratogenic-free drug. But it is also true that we have much more data on lithium and pregnancy than with any other drugs we use, so psychiatrists are able to better manage lithium during pregnancy and better inform their patients.

Other people may criticise lithium for being "not safe". Do you want to compare it to flashy newer drugs? Do you want to bet on its safety profile? Lithium, when is properly prescribed by a psychiatrist, is a safe drug. And let's not forget its antisuicidal properties.

The only problem I see with lithium is that it does not work unless the tablets are swallowed. It does not work from your pocket or from your medicine box. Lack of adherence or patients' refusal to take the prescribed medication is a major issue in bipolar disorder. Up to 40% of people affected by bipolar disorder do not take their medication as prescribed. Of course, lithium is not an exception; less than 10% of patients on lithium take it at least 90% of the time, which means that the vast majority of users take lithium irregularly. And this may lead to poor efficacy and to important side effects. Remember that lithium cannot help unless taken with regularity, but it may cause side effects even if it's only taken every now and then. When people suffering from bipolar disorder are asked about the major concerns regarding medication intake, the vast majority will answer by mentioning reasons having to do with lack of information, prejudice or myths regarding psychopharmacological agents. Patients' education becomes crucial. At the end of the day, who on earth would take a tablet without knowing its effects beforehand? It has been proven that those patients that have been properly educated regarding their treatments take their lithium more regularly, have more stable lithium serum levels and benefit more from the treatment. In other words, education stabilises the mood stabiliser.

Psychoeducative programmes are nowadays part of the treatment routines of every bipolar clinic and are acknowledged by each and every guideline. Psychiatry has left far behind the nonsense confrontation between psychotherapy and pharmacotherapy, and a major step has been made from a useless clash of paradigms to a profitable evidence-based synergy.

Dr John Cade himself, an advocate of biological psychiatry, started implementing group therapy as soon as he was appointed Superintendent and Dean of the clinical school at Royal Park Hospital, in Victoria, in 1952. This fact, per se, is an excellent example of the integrative approach that we all (should) use today.

I am grateful to Dr. Nick Stafford for allowing me to write the foreword to this very comprehensive book. I have been advocating for the need of high-quality and plain-written information targeted to people affected by psychiatric disorders for the last twenty years of my life and I consider this kind of initiative a major milestone in the way psychiatric disorders are perceived both by users, professionals, mass media and general public.

This book makes all the knowledge of psychiatry regarding lithium available and accessible to non-specialists. This is a must have for those who take lithium, their friends and caregivers. But it is also a wonderful book for psychologists, nurses, general practitioners and other non-psychiatrists medical doctors, as it summarises the available evidence and practicalities of the use of lithium.

We hope it will help with the myths and prejudice of bipolar disorder.

In the beginning there was lithium. A natural salt helping millions of people working hard to control their illness.

"Let's drink to the hard working people. Let's drink to the salt of the earth".

Dr Francesc Colom

Chapter One

What is Lithium?

The benefits of lithium

Lithium is the most established and widely used drug in bipolar disorder. It is used primarily as a mood stabiliser and antimanic agent but has other interesting properties. It has some antidepressant effects and a well recognised ability to significantly reduce suicide risk. Finally lithium is also has anti-aggression and dementia preventing properties.

The Benefits of Lithium

- Mood stabiliser
- Antidepressant
- Antimanic
- Suicide protection

Lithium is a metal

Lithium is a metallic element. It is the lightest of all the metals and is chemically similar to sodium and potassium. In its pharmaceutical tablet form it exists as a carbonate or citrate salt. As an element it is reactive to oxygen and its shiny metallic colour is usually covered in a white layer due to its reaction with air.

It is found in certain stones, hence the name lithium which comes from the Greek 'lithos' meaning stone. It is a very natural substance, being one of the first three elements in the universe to be created after the Big Bang some 14 billion years ago. It is present in some stars. If these stars are near a black hole the lithium in them is drawn to the surface by the intense gravity. This can be observed on earth, billions of light years away by the colour of its emanating light.

The history of lithium

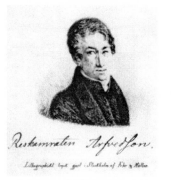

Johan August Arfwedson

Lithium was first discovered in 1800 as a compound substance called petalite by a Brazilian chemist on a small Swedish island.

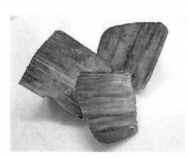

Lithium in its metallic form

However lithium was discovered as an element in its pure form by a Swedish chemistry student named Johan August Arfwedson (above) in 1817 working on the petalite ore. One year later it was found to burn with a characteristic red flame. In 1821, it was isolated as a pure element from solution using electrically charged plates placed in the fluid (known as electrolysis).

It wasn't until 1948 that an Australian psychiatrist named Dr John Cade discovered its effects as a mood stabiliser for bipolar. His experiments started by injecting the urine of mentally unwell patients into guinea pigs. He noticed that the guinea pigs injected by urine from the mentally unwell died sooner than those injected by urine from healthy people.

In an attempt to rectify this he added lithium to the urine in the belief that it would stabilise the solubility of the urea. As a result, he found that the toxicity of the urine was greatly reduced. He then realised that it was the lithium itself, rather than the effect on the urea that was the cause of the therapeutic effect. He initially tested the lithium on himself and then later performed trials on his manic patients, and his results were impressive. His work was marked by the side effects of lithium and some deaths in his patients due to toxicity. The regular use of lithium was then delayed by the development of a suitable test to measure the level of the lithium in the blood.

Studies have found that when lithium is present in higher concentrations in drinking water both the suicide and crime rates in that area are lower when compared to areas where the lithium concentrations are lower.

How lithium is used in other things

Lithium does not appear to have an essential function in any known living processes although it is found in trace amounts in most life forms. This seems odd since it has been around since the beginning of time, about 10 seconds after the Big Bang to be precise, which would lead you to believe that the evolution of life would have found some role for it.

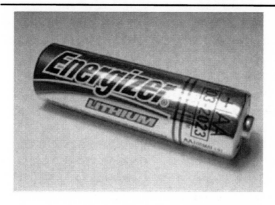

Energizer lithium
battery

Lithium has a number of other uses in physics and chemistry. When combined with some substances it renders them able to withstand high temperatures. It is used in aircraft engine components and high temperature greases and glasses.

It is also used in the production of nuclear weapons since it produces nuclear fuel when exposed to radiation. In chemistry, it is used to help stabilise reactions. It used to be added to the soft drink 7-UP and some beers in the USA in the belief it had medicinal properties. It was later removed as people suffered toxicity from it. Its most common use today is in lithium batteries found in many everyday electrical products.

Chapter Summary

Lithium is a metal salt whose beneficial properties in bipolar disorder were discovered over 50 years ago.

It has shown to be of benefit in the following ways:
- Anti-manic
- Antidepressant
- Mood stabiliser
- Protector against suicide

References

Mineral Information Institute, www.mii.org

Grunze H et al. World Federation of Societies of Biological Psychiatry (WFSBP)
guidelines for the biological treatment of bipolar disorders,
part III: Maintenance treatment.
The World Journal of Biological Psychiatry 5: 120-135, 2010.

Grunze H et al. World Federation of Societies of Biological Psychiatry (WFSBP)
guidelines for biological treatment of bipolar disorders,
part II: Treatment of mania.
The World Journal of Biological Psychiatry 4: 5-13, 2010.

Grunze H et al. World Federation of Societies of Biological Psychiatry (WFSBP)
guidelines for the biological treatment of bipolar disorders:
update on the Treatment of Acute Bipolar Depression.
The World Journal of Biological Psychiatry 1: 81-109, 2010.

Martín EL et al. High lithium abundance in the secondary of the black-hole binary
system. Nature 09 July 1992; 358, 129-131.

Chapter Two

How Lithium Works in the Brain and Body

We know that lithium works as a mood stabiliser (also known as 'maintenance' treatment), treating both depression and mania and that it also reduces the risk of suicide. We do not fully understand how it does this but our knowledge about it is growing all the time.

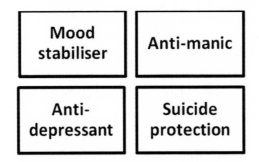

The clinical effects of lithium in bipolar disorder

Lithium works in bipolar on a number of levels: It has a direct effect on brain chemicals; it affects how cells send messages around themselves; it changes the level of brain hormones that stimulate brain cell growth; and it affects how genes work that control repair to the cells.

Let us consider these in turn.

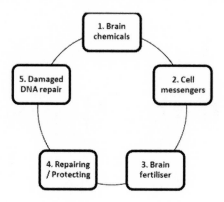

The five main ways we think lithium
works on the electronics of the brain

The effect of lithium on brain chemicals

When it comes to brain chemical levels, lithium is known to raise
levels of a number of 'feel good chemicals' known to help
depression including serotonin.

Lithium and its effect on the cell messenger system

Brain cells communicate with each other and also within themselves
using chemicals so that they can live, grow, divide and eventually
die. There are many ways cells communicate within themselves. One
of these is by using chemical switches that we call messengers.
Lithium affects a whole series of important messengers. Many of
these are involved in cell processes of cell resilience and
regeneration. Collectively these processes are called brain cell
plasticity.

The effect of lithium on brain fertilisers

Lithium increases the levels of brain fertiliser hormones. One of the main fertilisers is a substance called BDNF (whose full name is Brain Derived Neurotrophic Factor). BDNF is thought to help brain cells grow. In bipolar, BDNF repairs damage in affected areas of the brain, such as the mood thermostat circuits between the amygdala (the emotional powerhouse) and the prefrontal cortex (the executive controller of the amygdala).

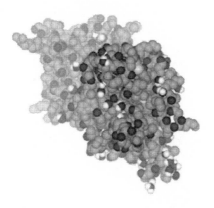

The BDNF molecule (brian derived neurotrophic factor)

Lithium on repairing and protecting the structures of the brain

The amygdala is the part of the brain that generates emotions very rapidly. It does this almost instantly, especially in evocative situations. It is the evolutionary centre that protects us against things that we have learned to fear. It also focuses on the things that we find pleasurable.

As we know, reacting to our raw emotions all the time is not usually helpful in a polite and civilised society. So the more evolved frontal area of the brain, known as the prefrontal cortex, acts as the executive management centre to regulate these strong impulses.

By using brain scans we can see that some people with bipolar disorder have unusually large amygdalae and a small prefrontal cortex. Not all studies have shown a reduced size prefrontal cortex.

Special brain scans that can see brain activity (functional brain images) also appear to show a problem with the circuits connecting the two structures. It is thought that lithium helps correct and protect this brain circuit. This circuit acts as a 'mood thermostat' by moderating the sensitivity, intensity and fluctuations of mood according to the environment.

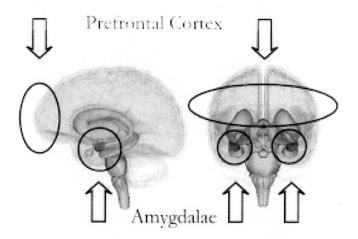

Side and front views of the brain showing the
position of the amygdalae and prefrontal cortex

In a similar way to this a thermostat controls the temperature of a house. If the thermostat is faulty the mood it normally controls becomes erratic.

Lithium affects the way genes are read and how proteins are manufactured

Genes are the code of life. They are the blueprints used to manufacture proteins making up almost all of what we are. Special proteins are used to read and process genes in the manufacture of other proteins. Lithium affects a number of proteins that are involved in this. In this way lithium can impact on the way certain genes are read, so causing brain cells to stay alive for longer and be more resilient in times of stress.

What happens to lithium tablets when you swallow them?

Once the lithium tablet is swallowed (ingestion) it passes down the oesophagus (food pipe) and enters the stomach where it dissolves and begins to enter the blood stream (absorption) as it passes into the duodenum, the next part of the intestines. Blood levels reach maximum levels about 2 to 4 hours after swallowing and slightly longer if the tablet is sustained release (this is the distribution phase). Lithium is then removed from the body by the kidneys (this

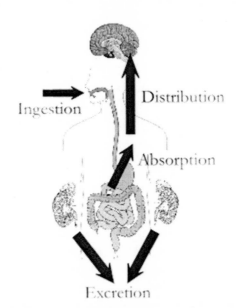

What happens to lithium when it is swallowed

is called excretion) at a rate that removes half of it from the body every 22 hours (known as the half life). It is distributed very broadly in the body and is dissolved freely in the blood and other body tissues. It slowly penetrates the blood brain barrier (the cells that protect the brain from toxins in the blood) and enters the brain and its surrounding fluid, the cerebrospinal fluid (CSF). Its levels in the CSF are less than half compared to the blood.

95% of the lithium you swallow is eliminated in your urine. The kidney exchanges sodium salt ions to excrete lithium and so any decrease in sodium increases lithium retention (blood levels rise). Likewise any increase in sodium can decrease lithium retention (blood levels drop).

The parts of the kidney responsible for lithium excretion are called the glomerulus and proximal renal tubule. Drugs which affect this part of the kidney can reduce lithium excretion and cause potentially dangerous increases in plasma levels.

These drugs include:
- Thiazide diuretics (water tablets) such as bendroflumethi-azide

- Nonsteroidal anti-inflammatory drugs (NSAIDS pain killers) such as aspirin, ibuprofen, diclofenac and mefenamic acid

- ACE inhibitors (for high blood pressure, heart failure, dia-betic neuropathy and kidney disease) such as benazepril, captopril, enalapril, fosinopril, lisinopril, moexipril, perindo-pril, quinapril, ramipril and trandolapril.

Are there any differences in how lithium is used in the body between racial groups?

The short answer to this, for lithium, is there are no differences. Nobody has found differences in the way lithium is absorbed and distributed in the body in different racial groups. The manner in which the gut absorbs the lithium, how it is distributed around the body and how the kidneys excrete it are all the same in different ra-cial groups.

This is not the case with more complex drugs that require the liver to metabolise them, such as anti-epileptics and antipsychotics. In these cases there can be a significant difference between races.

Chapter Summary

The way lithium works in bipolar is not completely understood. However there are a number of known mechanisms that are important. These include its effects on the following brain functions:

- Brain chemicals
- Cell messengers
- Brain fertilisers
- Repairing and protecting
- Damaged DNA repair

After lithium is swallowed it is absorbed and distributed throughout the body and then excreted. If its excretion is affected by other drugs the blood level of lithium may change.

References

www.Pharmacorama.com

Altshuler LL et al. Amygdala enlargement in bipolar disorder and hippocampal reduction in schizophrenia: an MRI study demonstrating neuroanatomic specificity. Archives of General Psychiatry. 1998 Jul;55(7):663-4.

Brambilla P et al. Anatomical MRI study of subgenual prefrontal cortex in bipolar and unipolar subjects. Neuropsychopharmacology. 2002 Nov;27(5):792-9.

de Sousa RT et al. Lithium increases plasma brain-derived neurotrophic factor in acute bipolar mania: A preliminary 4-week study. Neuroscience Letters. 2011 Apr 20;494(1):54-6. Epub 2011 Mar 6.

Lenox RH, Hahn CG. Overview of the mechanism of action of lithium in the brain: fifty-year update. Journal of Clinical Psychiatry. 2000;61 Suppl 9:5-15.

Lenox RH, Wang LE. Molecular basis of lithium action: integration of lithium-responsive signaling and gene expression networks. Molecular Psychiatry 2003. 8. 135–144.

Price LH et al. Lithium and serotonin function: implications for the serotonin hypothesis of depression. Psychopharmacology (Berl). 1990;100(1):3-12.

Salinas PC, Hall AC. Lithium and synaptic plasticity. Bipolar Disorders. 1999 Dec;1(2):87-90.

Sharma V et al. An MRI study of subgenual prefrontal cortex in patients with familial and non-familial bipolar I disorder. Journal of Affective Disorders. 2003 Nov;77(2):167-71.

Strakowski1 SM et al. The functional neuroanatomy of bipolar disorder: a review of neuroimaging findings. Molecular Psychiatry (2005) 10, 105–116.

Usher J et al. Correlation between amygdala volume and age in bipolar disorder - a systematic review and meta-analysis of structural MRI studies. Psychiatry Res. 2010 Apr 30;182(1):1-8. Epub 2010 Mar 11.

Chapter Three

The Clinical Evidence that Lithium Works In Bipolar Disorder

The scientific evidence supporting the benefits of lithium in treating bipolar disorder go back over 50 years and is both abundant and convincing. For the most part the evidence comes from studies in clinical research in which lithium is given to people with bipolar disorder under certain symptomatic states (depressed, manic, stable etc) and then comparing their response to a similar group of people who have been given a different drug or a placebo (a drug that looks like a drug but in fact has no active ingredient, like a sugar pill). These are called randomised controlled trails, or RCTs for short. This evidence from RCTs is reviewed here with lithium acting as:

- As an anti-manic drug

- As a mood stabiliser or maintenance drug

- As an antidepressant

- As a protector against suicide

The terms we use to describe phases of bipolar disorder

Bipolar disorder is characterised by a number of phases and we use specific terms to describe how treatment impacts on these phases. These terms are response, remission, recovery and relapse. These terms can apply to all phases of the illness such as mania, hypomania, depression, mixed state and so on. The terms are defined clearly so that clinicians and researchers have a common language when they talk about how treatments affect the illness. They are defined as follows:

- Response - if the symptoms of an illness phase are reduced by 50% or more by the given treatment. A symptom, such as mania, has a well validated and trusted scale to measure its severity, in this case the Young Mania Rating Scale (YMRS). The YMRS measures how severe the various symptoms of a person's illness are. So by example most research shows mania responds to lithium within 7 days of starting treatment. This means that when given at the right dose lithium will reduce the severity of mania as measured by the YMRS by 50% or more. Response is not the same as treating all of the symptoms.

- Remission is defined as an almost complete absence of symptoms of an illness phase. With mania this means that the condition is treated to remission by lithium after some weeks. Using the YMRS this means its score will be very low.

- Recovery is defined as a period of remission for a period of time, usually about 8 weeks.

- Relapse is a return of the symptoms of the illness. This is usually measured by a rating scale like the YMRS as above. In clinical practice relapse is usually defined on clinical assessment with the patient.

Lithium as an antimanic drug

More than 20 drug trials since 1954 demonstrate the ability of lithium to control a manic episode.

Antipsychotics (like olanzapine, risperidone and quetiapine) are also used to treat mania. Lithium is as effective as these in treating mania but not as fast acting as these drugs. Antipsychotics usually take about two days to have a significant effect on mania, whereas lithium may take up to a week. As a result lithium is usually used in combination with them. By combining these drugs with lithium their effectiveness in treating mania is boosted to around 125% compared to using lithium alone. Thus the combination is considered to be quicker, better and more significant.

Lithium as a mood-stabiliser

Studies comparing lithium to placebos have consistently shown that lithium reduces the chance of a mood relapse into mania or depression in bipolar disorder. There are many clinical trials and a number of reviews of studies on lithium that show lithium is more effective than placebo in preventing relapses of mood swing into mania or depression. This effect is clearer and stronger in preventing relapse into mania though it also works in preventing depression.

Furthermore, lithium is more effective if combined with another drug that has mood stabilising properties. In this way it is most commonly used with valproate.

The graph below shows how lithium, valproate and their combination can prevent a mood relapse in bipolar. The highest of the three lines represents valproate as a single therapy in mood stabilisation or maintenance. The vertical axis is the 'event rate', e.g. 0.8=80% relapse into hypomania, mania or depression. The horizontal axis tells us the time to relapse. And so the higher the line, the less effective over time that particular drug is as a maintenance drug for bipolar. The middle line represents lithium, and in this trial was found to be more effective than valproate.

However when the treatments are combined, seen in the lower line, one can see that this is the most effective outcome.

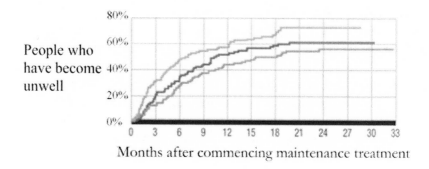

People who have become unwell

Months after commencing maintenance treatment

Relapse rate of bipolar disorder with valproate (top line), lithium (middle line) and both (lower line). From the BALANCE study, Lancet, January 30, 2010

Comparative studies with other mood stabilisers

Lithium has been compared to many other maintenance drugs and psychotherapy. Lithium is superior in many ways to most of these. Studies have shown that lithium is also well tolerated compared to most other drugs. These studies have looked at the following drugs:

Generic name	UK Trade Name
Aripiprazole	Abilify
Carbamazepine	Tegretol
Lamotrigine	Lamictal
Olanzapine	Zyprexa
Quetiapine	Seroquel
Semisodium valproate	Depakote

Lithium compared to carbamazepine

One study of 94 patients has shown that lithium is superior to carbamazepine in preventing relapse in bipolar disorder over a 2 year period. However, with the exception of an increased appetite, people taking lithium in the study had more side effects (see table below).

Adverse event	Lithium	Carbamazepine
Difficulty concentrating	45	33
Thirst	41	22
Hand tremor	31	4
Blurred vision	26	11
Reduced appetite	21	9
Increased appetite	17	33
Weakness	14	4

Lithium compared to valproate

Valproate comes in a number of formulations with different names including divalproex, valproate and semisodium. One twelve-month trial comparing lithium with valproate and a placebo showed there was no difference between lithium, valproate and the placebo in clinical outcomes. A study looking at hospital stay for all bipolar patients found no difference in hospital stay between people on lithium or valproate. There is some evidence that valproate is quicker at treating mania than lithium and that it is better in treating someone with mania who has had previous episodes. Another study showed that lithium was superior to valproate in preventing suicides.

Lithium compared to lamotrigine

Lamotrigine is an antiepileptic drug that has mood stabilising properties in bipolar disorder. It has an antidepressant effect, particularly when given with lithium. Its effects are quite weak and it doesn't seem to be that effective in preventing manic relapses. Some international guidelines such as CANMAT, the Canadian Network for Mood and Anxiety Treatments, recommend lamotrigine as a first line treatment in long term treatment to prevent depressive relapse.

Lamotrigine can cause serious skin reactions and in order to prevent these your doctor will need to increase its dose slowly. Too fast an increase in dose can lead to rare and serious rashes (called Stevens-Johnson syndrome). Unfortunately this means it can take weeks or months to get you to an effective dose to treat your depression effectively. It may therefore be better used as a relapse prevention drug rather than in an acute depression.

Lithium compared to olanzapine

Like lithium, olanzapine works well as a mood stabiliser in preventing manic episodes but probably not at all in preventing depressive episodes. It is probably better than lithium at preventing manic relapse and is also quicker to act. Lithium is better than olanzapine at preventing depressive relapse. Combining lithium with olanzapine in treating mania makes it more effective (by about 25%). Lithium is better in preventing either manic or depressive relapses if it is combined with another mood stabiliser. Finally lithium alone causes less weight gain than olanzapine alone.

Lithium compared to quetiapine

Quetiapine is an effective mood stabiliser in bipolar disorder. It works faster in the treatment of mania than lithium. It is different from other antipsychotics in that there is evidence that it is effective as an antidepressant in bipolar depression. This is useful as current evidence shows standard antidepressants are either ineffective or potentially harmful in bipolar depression.

Quetiapine is most effective in improving long term outcomes of bipolar disorder when combined with lithium or valproate. As already mentioned, lithium is a useful treatment in bipolar depression but can take a long time to work. Quetiapine however is both effective and shows clinically measurable improvement in bipolar depression by 2 weeks. Unfortunately quetiapine probably causes more weight gain than lithium.

Lithium compared to valproate

Lithium is more effective as a mood stabiliser in preventing both manic and depressive relapse in the long term when compared to valproate. However when combined with valproate (as described earlier in the BALANCE Study) the combination is more effective in preventing relapse than on its own.

Lithium compared to aripiprazole

Aripiprazole is effective at treating a manic or hypomanic episode and does this faster than lithium. Evidence shows that aripiprazole starts to work within 2 days as compared to lithium that works within 7 days. Aripiprazole is also an effective mood stabiliser, or maintenance treatment, in bipolar disorder. Studies following bipolar patients over a period of 2 years have shown that it is effective in reducing a mood relapse compared to a placebo, and as effective as lithium. As with lithium, it appears to be more effective in preventing manic relapses and less effective at preventing depressive relapses.

Lithium as an antidepressant

As mentioned earlier lithium has been shown to prevent relapse in bipolar disorder but it is less effective as an antidepressant. This is partly because bipolar depression is difficult to treat and can be resistant to many other drugs. However lithium is better at preventing a depressive relapse than a placebo and is better at doing this when combined with other drugs such as lamotrigine and some antipsychotics. Furthermore it lowers the risk of suicide considerably.

Lithium as a protector against suicide

Over the years studies have demonstrated lithium's protective effect against suicide. Collectively, these studies show that this effect is not only significant, but also becomes stronger the longer you take it. It may be that if you take lithium for more than a year your risk of suicide is reduced to almost that of the general population. This is

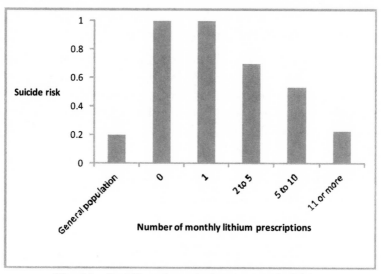

The risk of suicide reduces the longer you take lithium

an impressive statistic given that untreated bipolar disorder has a suicide rate of as much as twenty to thirty times the general population.

The graph on the previous page shows the risk of suicide as more lithium prescriptions are given. The risk of suicide for the general population is shown by the bar on the left hand side. By 11 or more prescriptions the risk of suicide is reduced to almost the same as the general population. The reason for this is unknown but may be a combination of mood stabilising, antidepressant and anti-aggression effects.

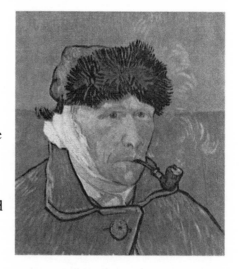

How long does it take for lithium to work?

The antimanic effects of lithium occur at higher doses than used for mood stabilisation and usually take around a week to show a significant effect. Lithium's mood stabilising effects are noticeable after a longer period of around 8 weeks. Lithium's antidepressant effect may take a few months. The antidepressant effect is quicker when used with other drugs, such as lamotrigine or quetiapine. As mentioned above, the full anti-suicidal effects of lithium can take up to a year to have full effect.

Chapter Summary

There is good clinical evidence that lithium acts well in all mood states in bipolar. It is also effective as a mood stabiliser but is better at preventing manic rather than depressive relapses. It is most effective in combination with other agents. It has a good side effect profile compared to other drugs used in bipolar. It is the most effective anti-suicidal agent for bipolar.

References

http://pn.psychiatryonline.org/content/45/5/13.full

Picture by Hendrike 2004, "Depression" Wikimedia Commons

Baldessarini RJ et al. Treating the suicidal patient with bipolar disorder. Reducing suicide risk with lithium. Annals of the New York Academy of Sciences. 2001 Apr;932:24-38; discussion 39-43.

Bowden CL et al. Efficacy of divalproex vs lithium and placebo in the treatment of mania. The Depakote Mania Study Group. JAMA. 1994 Mar 23-30;271(12):918-24.

Dalkilic A et al. Brief report. Effects of divalproex versus lithium on length of hospital stay among patients with bipolar disorder. 2000 American Psychiatric Association. Psychiatry Services 51:1184-1186, September.

Geddes JR et al. Lithium plus valproate combination therapy versus monotherapy for relapse prevention in bipolar I disorder (BALANCE): a randomised open-label trial. Lancet. 2010 375: 385-395

Goodwin FK et al. Suicide risk in bipolar disorder during treatment with lithium and divalproex. JAMA. 2003 Sep 17;290(11):1467-73.

Grunze H et al. World Federation of Societies of Biological Psychiatry (WFSBP) guidelines for biological treatment of bipolar disorders, part I: Treatment of bipolar depression. The World Journal of Biological Psychiatry 2010;11: 81-109

Grunze H et al. World Federation of Societies of Biological Psychiatry (WFSBP) guidelines for the biological treatment of bipolar disorders, part III: Maintenance treatment. The World Journal of Biological Psychiatry 2004;5:120-135

Hartong EG et al. LitCar Group. Prophylactic efficacy of lithium versus carbamazepine in treatment-naive bipolar patients. Journal of Clinical Psychiatry. 2003 Feb;64(2):144-51.

Herman E. Lamotrigine: a depression mood stabiliser. European Neuropsychopharmacology. 2004 May;14 Suppl 2:S89-93.

NICE clinical guideline 38 Bipolar disorder: the management of bipolar disorder in adults, children and adolescents, in primary and secondary care . National Institute for Health and Clinical Excellence. NHS. July 2006.

Revicki DA et al. Effectiveness and medical costs of divalproex versus lithium in the treatment of bipolar disorder: results of a naturalistic clinical trial. Journal of Affective Disorders 2005;86:183–93.

Rosack J. Lithium better than divalproex in keeping suicides down. American Psychiatric Association. Clinical & Research News. Psychiatric News November 7, 2003. 38(21):37.

Swann AC et al. Differential effect of number of previous episodes of affective disorder on response to lithium or divalproex in acute mania. American Journal of Psychiatry 1999 Aug; 156(8):1264-6

Yatham LN et al. World Federation of Societies of Biological Psychiatry Treatment Guidelines on Bipolar Disorders, World Federation of Societies of Biological Psychiatry (WFSBP) guidelines for biological treatment of bipolar disorders, part II: Treatment of mania. The World Journal of Biological Psychiatry 2009;4: 5-13

Yatham LN et al. Atypical antipsychotics for bipolar disorder. Psychiatric Clinics of North America. 2005 Jun;28(2):325-47.

Yatham LN, et al. Canadian Network for Mood and Anxiety Treatments (CANMAT) and International Society for Bipolar Disorders (ISBD) collaborative update of CANMAT guidelines for the management of patients with bipolar disorder: update 2009. Bipolar Disorders 11(3), May 2009; 225–255.

Chapter Four

The Side Effects of Lithium by How Common They Are

We will now review the side effects of lithium. Firstly these will be considered according to how common they are. The language we use of common, uncommon, rare and very rare side effects usually refer to the risks in the below table.

Table : What level of risk we mean by these terms?

Terminology	Incidence
Common	Greater than 10%
Uncommon	Between 1 and 10%
Rare	Between 0.1 and 1%
Very rare	Between 0.01 and 0.1%
Isolated reports	Less than 0.01%

These percentages mean that if 100 people take lithium:
- For 10% then at least 10 people out of 100 will experience the side effect
- For 1% then at least 1 person out of 100 will experience the side effect
- 0.1% means that at least 1 person in 1000 will experience the side effect

- 0.01% means that at least 1 person in 10,000 will experience the side effect

In the next chapter we will look at the side effects as they occur in different body systems, regardless of how common or rare they are.

Common side effects

Common side effects occur in 10% or more of the people taking lithium. Side effects in general may cause some people to stop taking it. Some side effects go away with time but some may persist for a long time. As with all drugs they affect different people in different ways therefore if someone you know has had bad side effects it doesn't mean you will. On the other hand just because they haven't does mean you won't.

Side effects are less common when the blood level is below 1.0mmol/L. Your doctor will usually try to keep your blood level between 0.6 and 0.8mmol/L. Most side effects are time limited to a few weeks. Most will improve with a slight reduction in dose.

Short term and dose related side effects	Long term side effects
Tummy upsets, tremor, unpleasant mood, fatigue, muscle weakness, unsteadiness, thirst, weeing a lot	Weight gain, weeing a lot, being very thirsty, thyroid problems

A study of 60 patients who took lithium for over 1 year (on average for 6.9 years) found the following percentages of common side effects. Note some side effects seem to occur more in men than women, or visa versa.

The table on the following page shows the percentage of people affected by side effects.

Side effects	Percentage affected
Drinking and passing too much urine	60%
Hypothyroidism in women	27%
Hypothyroidism in men	9%
Weight gain in women	47%
Weight gain in men	18%
Skin problems in women	16%
Skin problems in men	9%
Tremor in women	26%
Tremor in men	54%

Tremor

A fine hand tremor can occur and is more marked when you are tired or stressed. It becomes worse with focused movements. Some people find it socially embarrassing as it often occurs when holding a drink. In these cases it can be lessened by holding the drink with both hands. The tremor is not always present and tends to come

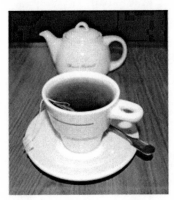

A cup of tea can be steadied with two hands if you have a tremor

and go. If it doesn't go away or is troublesome your doctor may be able to treat it with a beta-blocker drug like propranolol. If it spreads to other parts of the body you should see your doctor as it may mean you need to stop taking lithium.

The tremor may be caused by the lithium acting on areas of the brain regulating movement. At higher levels lithium has a toxic effect on these brain areas, movements become very coarse and walking can become difficult.

Thirst

Taking lithium can make you feel thirsty. The thirst can lead you to drink more sugary drinks which can be a common cause of weight gain when on lithium. Lithium makes the kidneys excrete more water to help get rid of it from the body. As a result you may go to the toilet more and get up in the night to pass urine. If this disrupts your sleeping pattern then you can lessen the problem by making sure you do not drink fluids for two hours before going to bed.

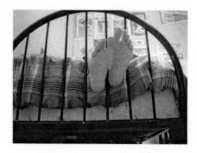

Nausea & Diarrhoea

Taking lithium tablets by themselves can cause nausea as they are rather chalky and hard to swallow. This can sometimes be avoided by switching to smaller tablets, such as from the 400mg to the 200mg. An upset stomach is a common problem with the lithium drug itself. This can cause nausea as well as bouts of the runs. The diarrhoea tends to be intermittent and made worse by fatty or spicy foods. It is not fully known why lithium causes intestinal problems but it may be because it interferes with the complex nervous system of the gut. We also know that emotional disorders, like bipolar, are often associated with gut problems such as irritable bowel syndrome.

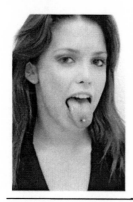

Metallic taste

Lithium can cause a metallic taste in the mouth especially at the start of treatment. This usually passes after a few weeks.
Lithium is a metal atom and so it is not surprising this happens. As with most tastes and smells that remain around us, we get used to it. It can be worse at higher doses or if your dose is increased.

Weight gain

Weight gain is common with lithium but should not be a problem if you take regular exercise and have a sensible diet. Part of the cause of the weight gain when you first start taking lithium could be a degree of water retention. Later there may be a change in your appetite which causes you to eat more or crave sugary and fatty foods. Also, as mentioned earlier lithium can make you more thirsty and you need to be careful not to drink too many sugary drinks.

Uncommon side effects

Uncommon side effects occur in between 1% and 10% of people taking lithium.

Fluid retention

Fluid retention, which can lead to water under the skin, causing things like swollen legs, may be caused by the effects of lithium on the kidneys. It affects the amount of urine produced and also the ability of the kidney to concentrate urine. Although this is common, it doesn't often cause significant weight gain.

Thyroid function

Lithium can cause the amount of thyroid hormone released from the thyroid gland to be reduced. This can lead to hypothyroidism (see under 'Thyroid').

Rare side effects

Rare side effects occur in between 1 in 10 and 1 in 100 people taking lithium.

Visual disturbance

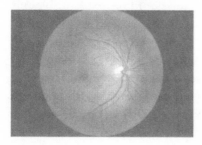

The human retina

Visual problems can occur but are rare with lithium. If the dose is too high it can cause blurred vision. In time it can cause loss of detail in your fine vision, or even small losses in your central vision (called scotomas). It may also cause problems with the vision in the corner of your eye (known as the peripheral vision). In all cases if you think your vision is affected you should contact your doctor immediately.

You may need to be assessed by a specialist eye doctor. Also, if you wear glasses or contact lenses you should always tell your optician that you take lithium, especially when you have your eyes tested for new glasses or lenses.

Skin rashes

Skin rashes may occur when you take lithium. If this occurs you should see your doctor immediately. It could indicate you are allergic to one of the components of the tablet. Allergy to the lithium itself does not occur. Alternatively you may be developing a serious skin reaction. Other skin complaints are less serious, can be troublesome but on the whole are rare. These include hair follicle inflammation (soreness and redness at the root of the hair), itching, skin papules (spots), acne, aggravation of psoriasis (a scaly thickening of the top skin layer), allergic rashes, alopecia (hair loss) and skin ulcers.

Tiredness

Tiredness rarely occurs with lithium. If it does occur, it probably means the dose is too high and will need reducing. If you experience this side effect then visit your doctor immediately.

Confusion

In more severe cases lithium can cause confusion. Again this tends to occur if the dose is too high and requires urgent medical attention.

Arrhythmia (an irregular heart beat)

If you get an irregularity of the heart beat (like missing beats), or it is too fast or too slow you will need a medical review. You may also feel faint, have chest pain or be short of breath. This may mean your lithium dose is too high but in any case you will need to seek an urgent medical opinion you may also need an ECG (the wiggly line produced by the electricity of the heart) as well.

Oedema (water retention)

Weight gain, severe swollen feet, ankles, face and stomach may be due to water retention with lithium. If it is severe or goes on for more than a couple of weeks you will need medical attention.

Your doctor should be very careful about prescribing diuretics or 'water tablets' for oedema of any cause as this can seriously affect the levels of lithium in your blood. Diuretics can make the level either too high causing a toxic reaction or too low and make the lithium ineffective. Frusemide is okay, with care, but the rest of the water tablets are not.

Cloudy urine

Cloudy or foamy urine is rare and may indicate a serious effect of the lithium on kidney function. This will require urgent medical attention.

Memory and creativity

Some people complain of memory problems. It is difficult to know if the bipolar disorder is the cause of this. Some in the artistic professions also complain that lithium affects their creativity. This is also difficult to prove and may be a direct cause of the bipolar process itself (see section on 'Creativity').

Fits or seizures

Fits are a rare and serious side effect and will require emergency medical attention. If this happens get yourself straight to hospital, by ambulance if necessary. Fits may/can be caused by a high level of lithium in the brain.

Very rare side-effects

Very rare side effects occur in less than 1 in 1000 people taking lithium.

High white blood cell count

Lithium can cause a high white blood cell count and this may last a long time. How lithium causes white cell production to increase is not known but is probably linked to its ability to reduce the usual death of blood cells (known as apoptosis, the programmed death of cells).

Raised calcium levels

Lithium can cause increased levels of calcium, magnesium and parathyroid hormone levels in the blood. These are all due to the effect lithium can have on the parathyroid glands, which are small glands that sit behind the thyroid gland in the neck that regulate the blood level of these substances.

Raised blood sugars

Raised blood sugars may occur, though why this is so is not understood. A possible cause is that with time, lithium can cause weight gain and this can make type II sugar diabetes more likely. However some studies have followed people taking lithium for years and found no raised glucose. It might therefore be a very rare and unpredictable reaction.

Benign intracranial hypertension

Benign (which means not harmful in effect) raised pressure in the head (benign intracranial hypertension, BIH) is a very rare side effect of lithium. Why this happens is not understood. It always resolves itself when the lithium is stopped. However there are complications after BIH, such as damage to the optic nerve.

Parkinson's Disease-like symptoms

Parkinson's Disease–like symptoms (like tremor, stiff muscles, difficulty walking and a mask-like face) are a very rare side effect of lithium. These are caused by the toxicity of lithium to certain brain areas that help control movement.

However some of the symptoms that are Parkinson's-like, such as a tremor are very common with other psychiatric drugs, in particular antipsychotics, especially risperidone and some of the older, first generation antipsychotics including haloperidol and chlorpromazine.

Chapter Summary

Everyone gets some side effects with lithium. Some side effects are common and others are rare. Not everyone gets the same side effects and many get better with time. Tell your doctor if you think you have side effects as some are important for them to know. Make sure you have your regular 3 monthly lithium blood tests. You should also have your renal function and thyroid function tested every six months.

References

The references for both chapters 4 and 5 are at the end of chapter 5.

Chapter Five

Side Effects of Lithium by Bodily System

Let us now consider each body system in detail and look at how lithium can affect them. These sections will be in more detail and may well repeat some earlier points.

Kidneys

Impaired kidney function

When lithium is taken over a long time (for at least 15 years) or at too high a dose the efficiency of the kidney in excreting waste products can become reduced in about 1 in 5 people (4 out 5 people are not affected). Some of these changes may be caused by becoming older and do not usually cause symptoms. This kidney function is measured in your regular blood test as eGFR and creatinine. eGFR stands for estimated glomerular filtration rate and is a measure of the kidney's ability to filter your blood of toxins before it concentrates your urine. If your eGFR is low (less than 50) you may need to see a kidney specialist. Creatinine is a measure of protein breakdown products which are partly removed by the kidney. If raised in the blood it indicates impaired kidney function.

Impaired renal function is more likely if lithium toxicity has occurred in the past. However if lithium levels are in the normal range those taking higher doses are not normally likely to develop problems. Men and women are equally affected and surprisingly the duration of treatment does not appear to increase the likelihood of reduced renal function if blood levels are in the normal range.

Diabetes insipidus

Diabetes insipidus is a form of kidney malfunction. It is caused by the kidney's inability to concentrate urine. Diabetes insipidus can be caused in two ways (see diagram). Firstly by direct damage to the kidney's urine concentrating systems (called nephrogenic diabetes insipidus) and secondly by its effect on the brain which releases a hormone called antidiuretic hormone (ADH) that in turn tells the kidney to concentrate urine. This is called hypothalamic diabetes insipidus.

Hypothalamic diabetes insipidus

ADH

Lithium

Nephrogenic diabetes insipidus

Lithium can cause diabetes insipidus by acting on the hypothalamus or kidney

However both nephrogenic and hypothalamic diabetes insipidus are reported in long term lithium use. Up to one in eight of people taking lithium may get diabetes insipidus of either type.

Other changes seen in long term lithium use as a result of kidney changes include high blood pressure and nephrotic syndrome (a change to the kidney structure that can cause them to leak protein). This is known as proteinuria, where protein is present in the urine. This should not happen as the kidney is impermeable to protein. In a small number of people this can cause end-stage renal failure, which unless treated by dialysis or transplant, will cause death.

The kidneys' ability to concentrate urine is reduced by lithium which leads to passing more urine. This affects between 1 in 5 and 1 in 2 of people on the drug. In time this usually becomes a permanent change. This effect may be improved by taking lithium once daily and in modified release formulation, the usual way lithium is taken in the evening.

A variety of changes to the cells, in a range of areas of the kidney are affected with long term use (greater than 5 years) and this can be seen under the microscope.

Renal failure

Renal failure is a rare side effect of lithium. When it happens it tends to do so after some years but can also occur in the early stages of taking it.

Though renal failure is rare, it is a serious complication and is one of the important reasons for close monitoring of lithium levels. It is more likely in people who have had periods of lithium toxicity and probably those who have taken it for longer periods; however it is not fully understood why it happens.

End stage renal failure (the final stages of kidney failure) is about six times more likely in those taking long term lithium than the general population. A study in Sweden found 18 people developed renal failure out of 3369 people who took it for an average time of 23 years (this is the same as 1 in 200 people).

Acute renal failure is marked by the passing of a very low volume of urine. In chronic renal failure this may not be noticed. It may take time for symptoms to become obvious in renal failure as toxins, such as urea, phosphate and potassium, accumulate in the body. High levels of urea in the blood can cause nausea, vomiting, diarrhoea, weight loss, weeing more (with pale urine), weeing less (with dark urine), blood in the urine and difficulty passing urine. High phosphate levels can cause bone damage and muscle cramps. High blood potassium can cause heart rhythm changes and muscle paralysis. Water retention may lead to swelling in the legs, ankles, face or hands. Shortness of breath may occur due to extra fluid on the lungs.

The kidneys are responsible for part of the pathway for producing red blood cells that are responsible for carrying oxygen in the blood. In renal failure less haemoglobin is produced and anaemia results. This can lead to tiredness and weakness.

If the filtering mechanism of the kidney is damaged and proteins are passed through (nephritic syndrome) the urine can become foamy or bubbly.

Heart

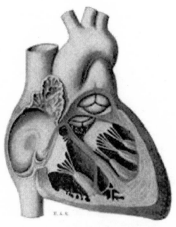

The human heart with the front wall removed revealing the internal valves

If you have a pre-existing problem with your heart you may still be able to take lithium, however any risks of side effects may be greater. All heart side effects of lithium are more likely if you are taking other drugs, psychiatric or otherwise, that affect the heart. Moreover if your blood lithium is higher you are more likely to get heart problems. The older you become the more these risks increase.

It is important to realise that people with bipolar disorder have an increased risk of heart disease in the first place. Heart attacks (myocardial infarctions), angina and high blood pressure are all more likely in bipolar disorder. This is probably due to the increased stress experienced in having the illness and a more likely possibility of smoking and other heart risk behaviours.

However lithium does not cause high blood pressure, even if it is taken for a long time. Very rarely it can cause low blood pressure after heart surgery.

The ECG (electrocardiogram) is the characteristic wavy lines on that machine the doctor wires to your chest. The lines are caused by the electrical activity of the heart. Lithium causes only small changes to various parts of the ECG. These changes are greater the higher the blood lithium level is.

Very rarely it may make the ECG trace look like a heart attack has occurred when it has not.

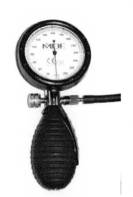

Lithium may very rarely cause an extreme slowing of the heart by affecting the part of the heart called the sinus node. This is the part of heart that acts as the natural pacemaker. In extreme cases this may cause the heart to go so slowly that collapse or death may occur. Lithium is most likely to be stopped if your heart slows in this way, alternatively you may require an artificial pacemaker to be fitted.

Even more rarely an increase in the heart rate (known as tachycardia) may occur if blood calcium is raised (another rare side effect of lithium). Studies have shown that the raised calcium is probably the critical factor in speeding up the heart rather than the lithium.

Sphygmomanometer

Very rarely lithium may damage the muscle of the heart, a condition known as cardiomyopathy.

Lungs

It is unlikely that lithium causes side effects in the lungs.

Ears, nose and throat

Lithium does not appear to cause side effects to ears, nose or throat.

Nervous system

The following side effects of lithium are very rare in the nervous system; they have been only occasionally reported:

- Myasthenia gravis – an autoimmune disease that leads to muscle weakness and fatigue
- Tingling or numbness of the skin
- Sleep walking
- Fits or seizures
- Confusion
- Reversible CJD (Creutzfeld-Jacob Disease)-like syndrome (like human mad cow disease)

Of course, all of these occur without lithium.

Overdoses in lithium can cause permanent nervous system damage. Movement, co-ordination problems and coma can last after lithium toxicity. Brain wave traces (EEG) commonly show changes when taking lithium. Many aspects of the EEG are affected but whether this is important is not fully understood.

There is no scientific proof that lithium can make you drive less safely but you must inform the DVLA if you are taking it. A study has shown that elderly people taking lithium were almost twice as likely to have a car accident although whether this was due to the lithium or their bipolar disorder could not be determined. However if you are not medicated and become unwell, either manic or depressed you certainly are more likely to have an accident.

The cerebellum is a part of the brain that helps co-ordinate movement and other brain activities. Very rarely lithium at normal blood levels can impair its function or cause it to shrink in size. In lithium toxicity when blood levels are greater than 2.0 or 3.0 mmol/l damage to the cerebellum becomes more common.

Damage to the cerebellum causes movement difficulties in that motor activity loses precision, producing erratic, uncoordinated, or incorrectly timed muscle movements.

There is a very rare nervous toxicity syndrome called SILENT (syndrome of irreversible lithium-induced neurotoxicity) in which irreversible damage to the brain including the cerebellum is reported. The lithium probably strips the nerve cells of their insulation so that they are no longer properly able to transmit

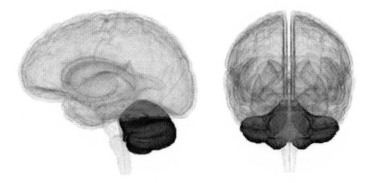

Cerebellum (shaded dark)

impulses. This sounds very scary but is extremely rare, so much so that only a few people in the world had ever had it.

Very rarely lithium can cause seizures of various types. This can occur at normal blood levels, high levels or if the drug is taken with other drugs that can cause fits as a side effect. It is likely that lithium reduces the 'fit threshold', a point at which the brain will have a seizure if stressed usually by a chemical imbalance. We all have a seizure threshold but a fit will only happen if yours is already low.

On a very rare occasion lithium has caused a reversible CJD-like syndrome. This is like the human form of mad cow disease and looks like a progressive dementia. The few cases that have occurred around the world have been associated with higher than usual blood lithium levels. It goes away when the lithium is stopped.

Parkinson's Disease symptoms occasionally occur in long-term lithium use. Symptoms can include a tremor, rigidity and restlessness. These symptoms are more likely if antipsychotics are or have been taken.

If lithium is taken with antipsychotics it can very rarely lead to neuroleptic malignant syndrome (NMS). NMS is a severe and life threatening reaction to psychiatric medication that leads to very high body temperature, rigidity of the muscles, delirium and blood pressure problems. It seems unlikely that lithium causes NMS by itself and that this problem is more linked to the antipsychotics.

A few cases of myasthenia gravis have occurred with lithium. Myasthenia causes muscle weakness and fatigue.

Benign intracranial hypertension (BIH) is a rare side effect of lithium and presents with headaches, reduced vision and a risk of blindness. If this occurs the lithium will have to be withdrawn and this usually corrects the problem.

Sleep walking has been found in some studies to be almost three times as common in those taking lithium. In the general population it occurs in about 1 in 40 and in those taking lithium it is almost 1 in 15.

Stuttering has been recorded very rarely. In one case it resolved when the person switched to another mood stabiliser.

Tremor is a common side effect of lithium. It can be made worse by:
- Tiredness
- Stress
- High lithium concentrations
- Caffeine
- Valproate
- Antidepressants
- A family history of tremors
- Being female

If troublesome the tremor can be lessened by reducing the dose of lithium or altering any of the above factors (like cutting down your caffeine). Some find it socially embarrassing, in particular when holding a drink in a glass or cup. A simple trick in these instances is to hold the cup with two hands, which cancels out the tremor. Other drugs, including those below, may reduce tremor, but may introduce other side effects:

- Beta-blockers such as propranolol, usually used in high blood pressure and also anxiety and panic attacks
- Primidone, an anti-epileptic drug
- Gabapentin, a drug developed to treat epilepsy but that is also used in pain and generalised anxiety
- Vitamin B6 which is found in foodstuffs (meats, whole grain products, vegetables, nuts and bananas) and amongst other things is needed in the manufacture of some brain chemicals

Skin

Lithium can cause a number of skin complaints. These are relatively common and reported in between 1 in 20 and 1 in 2 of people. They include:

1. Aggravation of psoriasis

2. Acne. This can be caused by or worsen with lithium

3. Inflammation of the hair roots

4. Maculopapular rash, a type of rash that has a flat, red area on the skin that is covered with small bumps

5. Darier's disease can be worsened. This is an inherited skin disease with dark crusty skin patches

Bones

There are no side effects on bones in those taking lithium. In fact one large study showed less likelihood of bone injury in those taking the drug.

Vision

Lithium can increase the sensitivity of the eyes to light. As a result bright lights and bright sun may cause damage to the retina. If your eyes feel more sensitive to light then you should protect them by removing yourself from the bright light or by wearing sun glasses.

Lithium may cause defects in fine central vision or peripheral vision (the corner of your eye). Specialist assessments by ophthalmologists can show whether this is the case. Specialised eye centres have high tech equipment that can look at the retina in fine detail and map your vision with accuracy.

Your ability to focus on close objects and reading may be affected only rarely. This also happen with increasing age so it is hard to tell if it is the lithium. Other rare effects include eyes movement problems.

Hearing

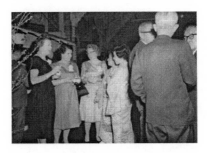

Tests on animals have shown that certain frequencies of sound, in particular lower frequencies, are reduced by lithium though these studies have not been done yet in humans.

A Cocktail party

The so-called 'Cocktail Party Effect' is the lack of ability to filter many different noises and focus on one particular noise, as in a noisy party when you are trying to focus on one person's voice. People with bipolar often complain this becomes a problem after they have developed the illness and it may also be a side effect of lithium.

Thinking Processes

Generally lithium does not appear to affect thinking processes. However mild effects are sometimes reported and it is not clear if this is an effect of the drug or the process of the illness itself. Bipolar is well known to cause certain thinking problems and interestingly these can also be seen in blood relatives of those with bipolar that do not have the illness.

Problems reported include:

- Reduced emotional reactivity in social situations. This makes you seem less animated in social situations, less 'tuned in' to the feelings of the other person.
- Reduced spontaneity
- Memory problems
- Finding it hard to choose words

- Longer reaction time
- Slowed speed of mental processing
- Impaired learning with repeated memory tasks. Usually people find it easier to learn when similar tasks a repeated. This may be affected when on lithium.
- Creativity (see 'Creativity' section)

It has been suggested that some of these effects may be caused by a low level of thyroid function that cannot be shown by usual tests. Taking a thyroid supplement may help. Another drug that may help (which is a food supplement in the USA) is aniracetam. It is a substance with anti-dementia properties but is not licensed in the UK.

Confusion, Delirium & Dementia

Lithium may help someone from getting dementia. It inhibits the effects of an enzyme (GSK-3) that usually leads to the formation of proteins that cause Alzheimer's disease. However having bipolar disorder by itself increases the chance of suffering Alzheimer's later in life and so taking lithium reduces this to about the same as the general population.

Lithium may make delirium (a serious mental confusion and altered level of consciousness) more likely but this isn't clear as some mood states in bipolar, in particular mania, can cause delirium and confusion.

Hair

Hair loss is rare although if thyroid function is affected the texture of hair can be affected. Treatment with thyroid hormone will correct this.

Immune system

Lithium by itself cannot cause an allergic reaction. However other components of the tablet or liquid may do so but only rarely.

Lithium can alter certain markers, proteins and cells in the immune system but none have been found to have a negative effect on immunity. In fact where white blood cells become depleted due to other drugs lithium is used to help increase their numbers.

Thyroid

Hypothyroidism (a low level of thyroid hormone) affects between 1 in 4 to 1 in 20 of people on lithium. This compares to 1 in 250 of women in the general population and 1 in 300 in men. In these cases the thyroid gland produces less thyroid hormone and the brain increases its output of thyroid stimulating hormone to try to counteract, but without effect.

This is a permanent change but can be easily treated by giving thyroid hormone replacement therapy known as levothyroxine.

Hypothyroidism can occur within weeks of starting lithium or it may take a number of years to develop.

One of the reasons this occurs is because lithium is taken up by in the thyroid gland and this reduces the released preformed hormone from the gland. It seems to interfere with the hormone packaging mechanism in the cells of the gland.

Thyroid gland

Parathyroid gland

The thyroid gland with the parathyroid glands sitting behind

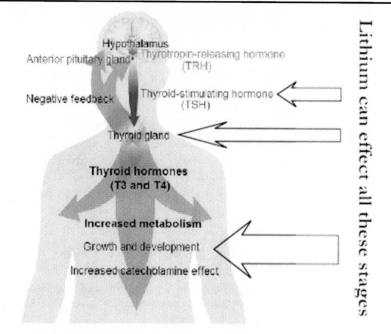

Symptoms of hypothyroidism include: feeling tired and sleeping a lot, feeling the cold easily, dry skin, coarse thinning hair, brittle nails, sore muscles, slow movements, a hoarse croaky voice, a change in facial expression, low mood, memory and concentration problems, weight gain and constipation.

Lithium can affect thyroid hormone in a variety of ways (see image on previous page):

1. Inhibiting its release from the thyroid gland
2. Blocking the action of the hormone (known as thyroid stimulating hormone / TSH) released from the brain which stimulates the thyroid to produce thyroxine
3. Increasing the breakdown of thyroid hormone in the body

The length of time you take lithium does not seem to make hypothyroidism more likely. However there is a chance that with each year you take it there is a increased chance you will experience thyroid problems year on year.

Those living in an area which is iodine deficient in food and water are more likely to have thyroid problems when taking lithium.

Rarely an increase in thyroid hormone can occur with lithium (hyperthyroidism or thyrotoxicosis). This happens in less than 1 in 100 of people on the drug and may be caused by an autoimmune reaction in the thyroid gland, something which may be a part of bipolar disorder, being made worse by the lithium. The treatment of thyrotoxicosis requires specialist treatment as you will need to be given drugs in careful doses to suppress the overactivity of the gland.

Symptoms of hyperthyroidism include: nervousness, irritability, being more emotional, tremor, sleep problems, intolerance to heat, weight loss with increased appetite, tiredness, weakness, raised heart rate, infrequent menstrual periods, more frequent bowel movements, shortness of breath, finer hair and hair loss, goitre (swollen thyroid gland) and swollen red eyes.
As many as half the people who take lithium can develop a swelling of the thyroid gland known as goitre. The number of people affected in this way is greater in areas where iodine is low in the diet, as iodine is essential for the thyroid gland to work properly.

Sexual side effects

Sexual side effects in men and women are very rare with lithium. Reduced libido, erectile problems and orgasm difficulty are only very occasionally reported. Other medication used in bipolar such as antidepressants and antipsychotics are much more likely to cause sexual problems. The mood states of bipolar, especially depression, are more likely to cause sexual problems, whereas mania can be disinhibiting.

Diabetes Mellitus

Type II diabetes mellitus (or sugar diabetes) is increased in bipolar disorder due to the stress of the illness and the less healthy lifestyle, on the whole, sufferers tend to lead. However there is no evidence that lithium itself increases this risk of developing diabetes mellitus.

Type II diabetes is a burn out of the insulin cells and an increased resistance to insulin in the rest of the body. It is not to be mistaken for diabetes insipidus which affects the kidneys (see 'Kidneys' and 'Diabetes insipidus').

Weight gain

Weight gain is a common side effect of lithium occurring in about 30-60% of people who experience an average increase of 4-7kg (8-15lbs). Higher doses of lithium make it more likely.

Why lithium causes weight gain is not fully known, however there are a number of possibilities. It may cause weight gain by slowing down the metabolism, the thyroid gland, increased consumption of sugary drinks, water retention and the effect of mood stabilisation impacting on diet. Many other drugs sometimes used with lithium are also responsible for weight gain such as antipsychotics and antidepressants. It is a common reason to stop taking lithium but can usually be managed effectively with diet and exercise.

The rate of obesity (being very overweight) is about one and a half times greater with lithium compared to the non-affected population. However those taking antipsychotics alone get an even greater rate of obesity of up to two and a half times the general population.

The risks of untreated bipolar

Whilst all these side effects of lithium can seem very scary it is important to recognise that untreated or poorly treated bipolar disorder is far more damaging to your health than all of these side effects.

Untreated bipolar not only causes extreme mental suffering and potentially suicide, but also significant physical health problems. Furthermore the uninhibited behaviour of hypomania causes you to take risk that can damage your relationships, your finances and you health.

Chapter Summary

Lithium can potentially affect many parts of the body, including the kidneys, heart, thyroid, nervous system, thinking processes and weight.

You would need to have various health tests done before starting to take lithium and then your blood levels and organ function should be tested on a regular basis. Keep a regular check on your weight.

References

Image attributions: http://www.flickr.com/photos/takomabibelot/496610682/
Photographers: Kevin Law; Purpleblue; TommyT

Internet resources:
www.bnf.org.uk
www.Bupa.co.uk
www.choiceandmedications.org.uk
www.drugs.com
www.emedicinehealth.com
www.mayoclinic.com
www.medicinenet.com
www.medicines.org.uk
www.nami.org
www.netdoctor.co.uk
www.rxlist.com

Alvarez-Cermeño JC. Lithium-Induced Headache. Headache: The Journal of Head and Face Pain. Apr 1989, 29, (4), p 246–247.

Ananth J et al. Lithium and memory: A review. The Canadian Journal of Psychiatry / La Revue canadienne de psychiatrie, May 1987, 32(4), p 312-316.

Andreasen NC et al. Bipolar affective disorder and creativity: Implications and clinical management. Comprehensive Psychiatry. May-Jun 1988, 29 (3), p 207-217.

Editor: Aronson JK et al. Meyer's Side Effects of Drugs, Fifteenth Edition: The International Encyclopedia of Adverse Drug Reactions and Interactions. Elsevier 2010.

Atmacaa M. Weight Gain and Serum Leptin Levels in Patients on Lithium Treatment. Neuropsychobiology 2002, 46, p 67-69

Baptista T. et al. Lithium and Body Weight Gain. Pharmacopsychiatry 1995, 28(2), p 35-44

Bendz H et al. Renal failure occurs in chronic lithium treatment but is uncommon. Kidney International. Feb 2010, 77(3), p 219-24.

Bocchetta A et al. The course of thyroid abnormalities during lithium treatment: a two-year follow-up study. Acta Psychiatrica Scandinavica. , Jul 1992, 86, (1), p 38–41.

Bocchetta A et al. Thyroid abnormalities during lithium treatment. Acta Psychiatrica Scandinavica. , Mar 1991, 83 (3), p 193–198.

Brust JCM et al. Acute generalized polyneuropathy accompanying lithium poisoning. Annals of Neurology 2004, 6(4), p 360-362.

Burrow GN et al. Effect of Lithium on Thyroid Function. The Journal of Clinical Endocrinology & Metabolism, May 1971 32 (5) p 647-652.

Callaway CL et al. Cutaneous Conditions Observed in Patients During Treatment with Lithium. American Journal of Psychiatry. Feb 1968. 124: p 1124-1125.

Chan HL et al. A control study of the cutaneous side effects of chronic lithium therapy. Journal of Affective Disorders. Jan-Mar 2000, 57, (1-3), p 107-113.

Chen Y et al. Lithium and weight gain. International Clinical Psychopharmacology, Jul 1990, Vol 5(3), p 217-225.

Christiansen C et al. Lithium, hypercalcemia, hypermagnesemia, and hyperparathyroidism. Lancet. 30 Oct 1976, 2(7992), p 969.

Conrad MS et al. Mitigating acute skin rashes and nausea from lithium. Comprehensive Psychiatry. 22 (3), May-June 1981, p 301-305.

Darbar D et al. Unmasking of Brugada Syndrome by Lithium. Circulation. Arrhythmia/Electrophysiology. 2005, 112, p 1527-1531

Engelsmann F et al. Lithium and memory: A long-term follow-up study. Journal of Clinical Psychopharmacology, Jun 1988, 8 (3), p 207-212.

Garland EJ. Weight gain with antidepressants and lithium. Journal of Clinical Psychopharmacology, Oct 1988, Vol 8 (5), p 323-330.

Gelenberg AJ et al. Lithium tremor. Journal of Clinical Psychiatry. 1995 Jul;56(7): p 283-7.

Gelenberg AJ et al. Comparison of Standard and Low Serum Levels of Lithium for Maintenance Treatment of Bipolar Disorder. New England Journal of Medicine. 1989. 321, p 1489-1493.

Gregoor PS et al. Lithium hypercalcemia, hyperparathyroidism, and cinacalcet. Kidney International. Mar 2007, 71(5), p 470.

Henry C. Lithium side-effects and predictors of hypothyroidism in patients with bipolar disorder: sex differences. Journal of Psychiatry Neuroscience. 2002 March; 27(2): p 104–107.

Honig A et al. Lithium induced cognitive side-effects in bipolar disorder: a qualitative analysis and implications for daily practice. International Clinical Psychopharmacology. May 1999, 14 (3).

Jamison KR. Mood disorders and patterns of creativity in British writers and artists. Psychiatry: Interpersonal and Biological Processes. 52(2), May 1989, p 125-134.

Jasleen G et al. Acute Lithium Intoxication and Neuroleptic Malignant Syndrome. The Journal of Human Pharmacology and Drug Therapy Pharmacotherapy. Jun 2003, 23 (6), p 811-815.

Judd LL et al. The Effect of Lithium Carbonate on the Cognitive Functions of Normal Subjects. Archives of General Psychiatry. 1977, 34(3), p 355-357.

Källén B et al. Lithium and pregnancy. A cohort study on manic-depressive women. Acta Psychiatrica Scandinavica. Aug 1983, 68 (2), p 134–139.

Kaplan PW et al. Lithium-induced Confusional States: Nonconvulsive Status Epilepticus or Triphasic Encephalopathy? Epilepsia. Dec 2006, 47 (12), p 2071–2074.

Kaufman PL et al. Ocular effects of oral lithium in humans. Acta Ophthalmologica. 1985, 63, (3), p 327–332.

Kinga JR et al. Side-effects of lithium at lower therapeutic levels: the significance of thirst. Psychological Medicine 1985, 15: p 355-361

Kusalic M. Effect of lithium maintenance therapy on thyroid and parathyroid function. Journal Psychiatry Neuroscience. May 1999; 24(3): p 227–233.

Kusumi Y. A cutaneous side effect of lithium: Report of two cases. Diseases of the Nervous System. Dec 1971, 32 (12), p 853-854.

Kusumo KS et al. Effects of lithium salts on memory. The British Journal of Psychiatry. 1977, 131, p 453-457.

Lapierre YD. Control of lithium tremor with propranolol. Canadian Medical Association Journal. 1976 April 3; 114(7): p 619-20, 624.

Lazarusa JH et al. Lithium therapy and thyroid function: a long-term study Psychological Medicine 1981, 11, p 85-92.

Lazarus JH et al. The Effects of Lithium Therapy on Thyroid and Thyrotropin-Releasing Hormone. Thyroid. Oct 1998, 8(10), p 909-913.

Lee S. Side effects of chronic lithium therapy in Hong Kong Chinese: an ethnopsychiatric perspective. Cultural Medical Psychiatry. 1993 Sep, 17(3), p 301-20.

Leroy M et al. Lithium, thyroid function and antithyroid antibodies. Progress in Neuro-Psychopharmacology and Biological Psychiatry. 1988, 12 (4), p 483-490.

Lydiard RB et al. Hazards and Adverse Effects of Lithium. Annual Review of Medicine. , 1982, 33, p 327-344.

Marshall MH et al. Psychosomatics. Lithium, creativity, and manic-depressive illness: review and prospectus. Sep-Oct 1970, 11(5), p 406-8.

Mellerup ET et al. Lithium, weight gain, and serum insulin in manic-depressive patients. Acta Psychiatrica Scandinavica. Aug 1972, 48, (4), p 332–336.

Murphy DL et al. Leukocytosis during lithium treatment. American Journal of Psychiatry. May 1971, 127(11), p 1559-61.

Murray L et al. Lithium associated thyrotoxicosis: a report of 14 cases, with statistical analysis of incidence. Clinical Endocrinology. Jun 1994, 40 (6), p 759–764.

Myersa DH et al. A prospective study of the effects of lithium on thyroid function and on the prevalence of antithyroid antibodies. Psychological Medicine 1985, 15: p 55-61

Oakley PW et al. Lithium: Thyroid Effects and Altered Renal Handling. Clinical Toxicology. 2000, 38 (3), p 333-337.

Penney MD et al. The effect of lithium therapy on arginine vasopressin secretion and thirst in man. Journal of Clinical Biochemistry 1990, 23 (2) p 233-236

Persson G. Lithium side effects in relation to dose and to levels and gradients of lithium in plasma. Acta Psychiatr Scand. 1977 Mar, 55(3), p 208-13.

Peselow ED et al. Lithium carbonate and weight gain. Journal of Affective Disorders. Dec 1980, 2 (4), p 303-310

Rifkin A et al. Lithium-Induced Folliculitis. American Journal of Psychiatry. , Sept 1973, 130: p 1018-1019.

Rolls BJ et al. Thirst. Cambridge University Press. 1982.

Rothenberg A. Bipolar illness, creativity, and treatment. Psychiatry Quarterly. Summer 2001, 72(2), p 131-47.

Schou M. Biology and pharmacology of the lithium ion. Pharmacological Reviews. March 1957, 9, p 17-58

Schou M. Artistic productivity and lithium prophylaxis in manic-depressive illness. British Journal of Psychiatry. Aug 1979, 135, p 97-103.

Shah AK et al. Case report: Acute confusional state secondary to a combination of fluoxetine and lithium. International Journal of Geriatric Psychiatry. Sept 1992, 7 (9), p 687–688.

Shaw ED et al. Effects of lithium carbonate on associative productivity and idiosyncrasy in bipolar outpatients. American Journal of Psychiatry. 1986, 143, p 1166-1169.

Shopsin B et al. Lithium and leukocytosis. Clinical Pharmacological Therapeutics. Nov-Dec 1971, 12(6), p 923-8.

Smith M. Van Gogh and lithium. Creativity and bipolar disorder: perspective of an academic psychologist. Australian and New Zealand Journal of Psychiatry. , Dec 1999, 33 Suppl, S120-2.
Sarantidis D et al. A review and controlled study of cutaneous conditions associated with lithium carbonate. The British Journal of Psychiatry. 1983 143, p 42-50.

Sharon Smaga MD. Tremor. American Family Physician. 2003 Oct 15;68(8): p 1545-1552.

Spaulding SW et al. The Inhibitory Effect of Lithium on Thyroid Hormone Release in Both Euthyroid and Thyrotoxic Patients. The Journal of Clinical Endocrinology & Metabolism 1 Dec 1972, 35 (6).

Squire LR et al. Effects of lithium carbonate on memory and other cognitive functions. American Journal of Psychiatry. 1980; 137: p 1042-1046.

Tangedahl TN. Myocardial Irritability Associated with Lithium Carbonate Therapy. New England Journal of Medicine. 26 Oct 1972, 287, p 867-869.

Tilkian AG et al. The cardiovascular effects of lithium in man: A review of the literature. The American Journal of Medicine Nov 1976, 61(5), p 665-670.

Tilkian AG et al. Symposium on Hypertension. The cardiovascular effects of lithium in man: A review of the literature. The American Journal of Medicine. Nov 1976, 61 (5), p 665-670.

Tilkian AG et al. Effect of lithium on cardiovascular performance: Report on extended ambulatory monitoring and exercise testing before and during lithium therapy. The American Journal of Cardiology. 23 Nov 1976, 38 (6), p 701-708.

Vestergaard P. et al. Acta Psychiatrica Scandinavica. Tremor, weight gain, diarrhea, psychological complaints. Prospective studies on a lithium cohort. 1988

Chapter Six

Special Issues With Lithium

Lithium toxicity

This is very rare but there can be serious consequences of the lithium level in the blood being too high (usually blood levels above 2.0mmol/L). The following side effects may be signs of lithium toxicity:

Gut symptoms

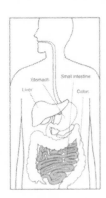

Loss of appetite, diarrhoea, vomiting and feeling very sick. As the lithium level rises in your blood there are special centres in your brain that become triggered. These centres detect the high level of lithium and assume that the toxic substance is coming from your gut and so triggers mechanisms to clear the gut out leading to problems at both ends of your intestines.

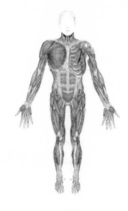

Muscles and movements

Muscle weakness, lack of coordination, muscle twitching, sudden jerks and shaking. High blood lithium levels cause an imbalance in the basic salt levels of cells in the body such as sodium and potassium. All of these changes make the muscles weaker, nerves work less well and parts of the brain to work poorly. In particular the cerebellum which controls coordination and movement timing is affected.

Concentration and attention

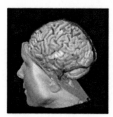

Feeling drowsy, very tired, balance problems and feeling dizzy with vertigo (a feeling of being dizzy as if on a high building). These are all symptoms caused by the high lithium levels in the blood crossing into the brain and causing a chemical imbalance making the brain very confused.

Movement

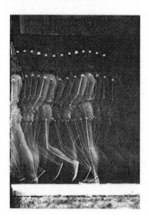

Difficulty walking, unusual voluntary movements of the limbs including unusual eye movements. As already mentioned the high levels of lithium can affect almost any cell in the body. There are a number of centres in the brain that control all kinds of muscles and movements in different body parts. Their function is reduced by high levels of lithium. They include the cerebellum, thalamus and colliculi.

Tinnitus and blurred vision

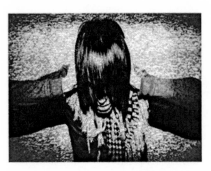

Tinnitus (ringing in the ears) rarely occurs at normal lithium levels. However when levels become toxic it becomes more frequent. It is caused by what is probably a direct toxic effect on the cells in the inner ear that detect sound. Similarly vision may become blurred due to the effect of a high lithium concentration on the muscles in the eyes.

Speech problems

Speech is a highly evolved and complex function that involves many areas of the brain and their proper connections. Just as high lithium levels can cause problems in movements such as walking, it is not surprising that more complex functions like speech are also affected. If this happens your speech becomes slurred, you may stutter and feels as if your thinking and words become mashed up.

IF YOU EXPERIENCE ONE OR ANY NUMBER OF THESE SYMPTOMS THEN ATTEND YOUR NEAREST A&E / EMERGENCY ROOM AS SOON AS POSSIBLE.

Death caused by lithium

Deaths caused by lithium are extremely rare and always caused by lithium toxicity (see above). When blood levels are greater than 2mmol/L this becomes increasingly likely.

It is important to recognise that death is less likely in people taking lithium compared to those taking other drugs since:

1. Lithium reduces the risk of suicide

2. The effects of some antipsychotics on the metabolism increase the risk of heart disease and stroke

3. People with bipolar who take lithium tend to better manage their overall health, diet and also exercise more

Pregnancy

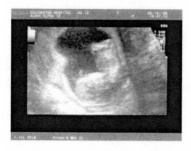

It used to be though that lithium should not be taken in pregnancy, especially the first 3 months (first trimester) of gestation, however it now is prescribed. Lithium can damage the development of the unborn child and cause congenital heart malformations, foetal and neonatal heart rhythm problems, low blood sugar, premature birth, and other adverse outcomes. The baby is formed very early on in the pregnancy and the heart in the first fourteen days. So if you are already on lithium it would be too late to stop it. However the risk of foetal damage must be weighed against the risk of relapse to the mother and the impact a relapse will have on her and the developing baby. Therefore stopping the drug would not usually be recommended.

Lithium passes freely through the placenta into the umbilical cord blood and then the unborn baby. It is also highly concentrated in the amniotic fluid in which the baby floats in the womb.

Until more recently the risk of heart defects was considered to be very high based on early studies. In the 1970s the lithium birth register of Denmark showed that the risk of a very rare heart defect called Ebstein's anomaly (which can be fatal) was raised from 1 in every 20,000 births to 1 in 50 births. However more recent and better controlled studies have put this increased risk at about 1 in 1000 to 2000 (0.05-0.1%). As a result more women are opting to stay on lithium during pregnancy but with closer monitoring of the unborn child by foetal ultrasound at 18-20 weeks. It should also be noted that the risk to the unborn child is much higher with sodium valproate and carbamazepine than with lithium.

Babies born to mothers whose blood lithium level was greater than about 0.6mmol/L are less responsive at birth and tend to stay longer in hospital after delivery. To date research also suggests that children born to mothers taking lithium develop normally.

In women who suffer with more severe frequent bipolar episodes, lithium is more likely to be continued, but with full counselling about the risks to the unborn child. Also the dose of lithium may be reduced, especially during the first trimester (the first 3 months) of the pregnancy.

As pregnancy affects the way the body handles lithium, close monitoring will be needed during pregnancy and after delivery to detect and prevent high blood levels.

It must also be remembered that semisodium valproate (and sodium valproate) is even more toxic to the unborn child with birth defects occurring in as many as 1 in 10 (10%) of babies born to women taking it. Children to born to mothers taking valproate also tend to have lower IQs and increased educational needs.

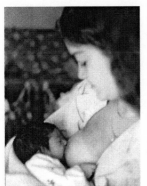

Various guidelines exist around the world on the use of lithium in pregnancy and they all say slightly different things. If you ask different specialists you are also likely to get different opinions. This is due to the relatively recent review of our knowledge of the risk of lithium to the unborn child and that changing prescribing habits in pregnancy in risky groups can be slow.

Breastfeeding

Enough lithium is excreted in the breast milk to affect your baby. Concentrations in the breast milk are about 40% of that in the blood.

The lithium in the breast milk can theoretically affect the newborn baby in a number of ways.

You will need to make a decision with your doctor as to whether you wish to continue lithium and not breastfeed or breastfeed and not take lithium.

Contraception

As far as is known lithium does not knowingly affect the female oral contraceptive pill. If you suffer sickness or diarrhoea as a result of taking lithium you will need to take additional contraceptive precautions. Also since lithium may cause damage to the unborn child a consultation with your doctor on reliable forms of contraception is essential.

Fertility

Lithium does not appear to affect the function of the ovaries or the menstrual cycle in women.

Creativity

Some people complain that lithium reduces their creative skills. There are many arguments about whether this is a true effect. There is more than one answer to this question and any or all of them could be correct. There is good evidence that there is a higher number of creative people with bipolar disorder than in the general population.

Professor Kay Redfield Jamison's book "Touched with Fire" provides a good analysis of creativity in bipolar.

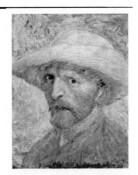

Of course, this does not mean that everyone with bipolar disorder is highly creative. Overall the impact of the illness, the long term effects of mood episodes and its impact on thinking abilities are probably more likely to affect any existing creative abilities.

It seems that the intense suffering and elation experienced in some bipolar sufferers may give rise to special insights which when coupled with the skills to express these creatively, the genius within those like Vincent van Gogh, Winston Churchill and Florence Nightingale are born.

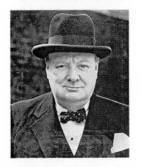

Proving whether lithium has a negative effect on creativity is difficult because creativity is hard to define and then measure scientifically. Creativity is a very broad and mixed concept. It is not like a symptom (or collection of symptoms like depression) which can be easily understood, although the field of psychology is developing scales and measures to do this.

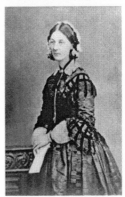

Despite these difficulties some people with bipolar disorder involved in creative professions do sometimes complain that lithium dulls their creativity. This could be for a number of reasons:

1. It is a true effect of the lithium
2. The dose of lithium could be too high

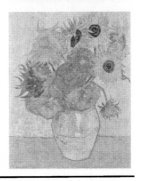

3. Their creativity could be affected by processes of the illness as bipolar does cause cognitive (thinking) deficits

4. The lithium could be successfully treating mania and this might lead to a relative feeling of dulled creativity

Any one or all of these could be true and there may be different effects for different people.

Are there any special warnings for other health conditions?

Age

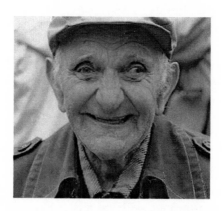

With increasing age it is likely that you can become more sensitive to many of the side effects of lithium. Closer medical monitoring of your physical health is important. In treating mania in older people many psychiatrists are less likely to use lithium in higher doses due to the various risks, which are worsened by the more fragile physical and mental state of someone suffering mania. They are more likely to use another agent like valproate or add an antipsychotic.

As you get older you are more likely to be prescribed other drugs as well as your lithium. It is important that your various physicians communicate well with each other so that you are not given a drug that interacts with your lithium (see list below).

Kidney function

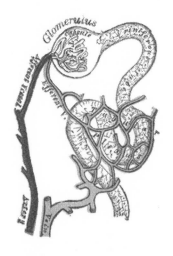

Lithium is excreted almost entirely by the kidney, so if your kidney function is impaired, care will need to be taken when you are prescribed lithium. Your dose may need to be lower and your blood monitoring more frequent. If your kidney function is severely impaired then you should not take lithium. It is possible lithium may damage kidney function if taken over many years but this is by no means certain as many people take it for long periods without difficulty.

Drawing of the filtering system of the kidney as seen under the microscope.

Fluid & salt balance

Your lithium blood levels need to be tested regularly during episodes of nausea, vomiting, diarrhoea, excess sweating or dieting. Drugs that affect the fluid balance such as diuretics (or water tablets) need to be prescribed with care. Severe infections may also affect fluid balance.

Fits

Lithium lowers the fit threshold of the brain but this only very rarely leads to fits. It does not tend to cause fits by itself but can cause seizures if given with other drugs that do likewise.

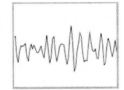

Benign intracranial hypertension (BIH)

Very rarely lithium can cause benign intracranial hypertension (a raised pressure in the head) which can lead to headaches and visual disturbances.

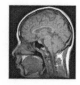

Heart rhythms

Lithium should be avoided in people with certain heart rhythm problems (QT prolongation & Brugada syndrome) as this can cause a fatal reaction.

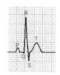

The dose of lithium

The dose depends on the form of lithium you take (usually around 400-1200mg per day), and your blood level. Normal blood levels also depend on the hospital or doctor you see, and the method the lab uses to do the test. The UK NICE Guidelines recommend between 0.6 and 0.8mmol/l. However the usual range is around 0.4 to 1.2 mmol/l.

What happens if I overdose on lithium?

If you are feeling suicidal you should speak to someone about it straight away. Talk to a loved one or someone you trust, your doctor or mental health professional.

If you do take an overdose of lithium you should attend casualty immediately, if necessary by ambulance. You will be closely monitored for a number of hours depending on the amount you have taken. You may need to have your stomach washed. If this is not enough you may need dialysis (a machine that washes your blood) to wash the lithium out of your blood.

How long will I take it?

It is probably best to take lithium for life. The longer you can take it the better. If you have to stop you will need to do so gradually as stopping too quickly may lead to a 'rebound mania'. At least 4 weeks to be safe but ideally over at least 3 months. Some doctors worry about giving it for too long because of the risk of kidney damage.

Will I become addicted to lithium?

No. But if you need to stop taking lithium it must be done slowly as stopping too quickly can cause a manic episode.

How often should my lithium be reviewed?

To start with your doctor will need you to have blood tests to check your kidney and thyroid levels, as well as an ECG. Whilst you are finding the right dose of lithium you may need blood tests every few weeks. Once settled on the right dose you will need blood tests every few months. In the UK according to the National Patient Safety Agency (NPSA), lithium levels should be taken every three months and kidney and thyroid levels every six months.

Driving whilst taking lithium

You can drive while taking lithium. However it may slow reaction times and so you should take care when driving or operating machinery. You must by law inform the DVLA (the UK driving regulatory authority) of your bipolar disorder and your lithium and they will decide your fitness to drive. After manic or depressive episodes and particularly after hospital admissions you may have your license revoked for a few months.

Can I drink alcohol?

You can drink alcohol, though only in moderation. It is believed that lithium may increase the effects of alcohol on the brain. Also excessive and regular alcohol intake is very destabilising to your mood.

Are there any foods or drinks I should avoid?

No. There are no known foods or drinks that interact with lithium.

What should I do if I forget to take a dose?

If it is less than twelve hours after the time you forgot your dose you should simply take the dose now. If more than twelve hours have elapsed since you missed your dose, simply skip the missed dose and start taking lithium from the next time you are due to take medication.

What will happen if I stop taking it suddenly?

Suddenly stopping lithium is unwise because you can suffer a severe rebound mania within weeks or months. It is better to come off lithium under the supervision of your doctor over a period of months. This should be done over at least a four week period of around three months if possible.

Will lithium interact with other medicines?

The level of lithium can increase if taken with the following drugs:

- Metronidazole
- NSAIDS (non-steroidal anti-inflammatory drugs) pain killers such as aspirin, ibuprofen, naproxen, mefenamic acid
- COX2 inhibitors such as etoricoxib and rofecoxib
- ACE inhibitors such as captopril, cilazapril, enalapril, fosinopril, imidapril, lisinopril, moexipril, perindopril, quinapril, ramipril and trandolapril
- Angiotensin II receptor antagonists
- Diuretics (water tablets), such as bendrofluazide and bumetanide
- Steroids such as prednisolone
- Tetracyclines

The level of lithium can decrease if taken with the following drugs:

- Xanthines (theophylline, caffeine)
- Sodium bicarbonate products, such as Rennies and other indigestion remedies
- Diuretics
- Urea

Though rare, some of the following drugs can cause toxicity to nerve and brain cells when taken with lithium:

- Antipsychotics (particularly haloperidol at higher doses)
- Flupenthixol
- Diazepam
- Thioridazine
- Fluphenazine

- Chlorpromazine
- Clozapine

These drugs may in rare cases lead to severe neurotoxicity (damage to brain cells) with symptoms such as confusion, disorientation, lethargy, tremor, extra-pyramidal symptoms and myoclonus (muscles becoming contracted). Increased lithium levels were present in some of the reported cases.

Stopping both drugs is recommended at the first signs of toxicity.

SSRI antidepressants can cause serotonin syndrome with lithium. This is caused by too high a concentration of serotonin building up in the brain. The symptoms of serotonin syndrome include agitation, confusion, unstable blood pressure and tremor.

Early signs of serotonin syndrome include tremor, restlessness and diarrhoea. Agitation, pressured speech and hypersensitivity may occur later. In severe cases delirium may occur.

Lithium must be given with care with other drugs that affect the heart ECG trace.

Does Lithium have more than one name?

Lithium comes in a variety of formulations whose brand names in the UK are: Priadel; Camcolit; Liskonium and Li-Liquid.

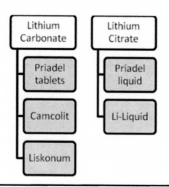

The trade names for lithium arranged according to whether they are lithium carbonate or citrate.

The brand name of lithium may vary in different countries.

Chapter Summary

It is important to know the symptoms of lithium toxicity and report them to your doctor immediately. Lithium can be used in pregnancy but you will need to assess the risks and benefits to the unborn child. A relapse of a bipolar illness in pregnancy is known to be damaging to the unborn child.

Creativity may be affected by lithium but this has not yet been proven. If you have existing health problems or are on other medication you may need special monitoring.

Chapter Seven

Lithium in Bipolar I, Bipolar II and Cyclothymia

Bipolar disorder is not a single illness that presents with the same symptoms in every person. It is a spectrum of related conditions that have at their heart mood swings which are characterised by elation and depression. The pattern, nature and degree of these mood swings are classified as bipolar I, bipolar II and cyclothymia.

The terms are:

- Bipolar I disorder: characterised by upward mood swings that are considered manic. Mania (as opposed to hypomania) is so severe it means that you are unable to function because of the degree of symptoms. In most cases if you are manic you will need to be in hospital.

- Bipolar II disorder: characterised by upward mood swings that are considered hypomanic. Hypomania is less severe than mania and does affect how you function. Other people notice you have symptoms but you are not so unwell as to need inpatient care.

- Cyclothymia: This is characterised by upswings in mood that are not severe enough or have the number or degree of symptoms to be defined as hypomania.

In summary bipolar I, bipolar II and cyclothymia represent different severities of upswings in mood. This does not mean that bipolar I is more severe than bipolar II and so on. Most people with bipolar disorder of any type spend most of their time suffering from bipolar depression. Bipolar depression is certainly as severe in both bipolar I and II disorder and is probably as disabling in cyclothymia in some cases.

The differences between these can be shown in the graphs below:

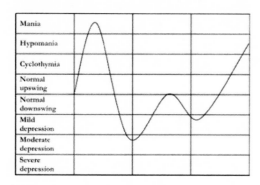

Bipolar I mood swings

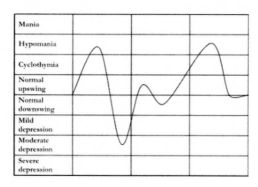

Bipolar II mood swings

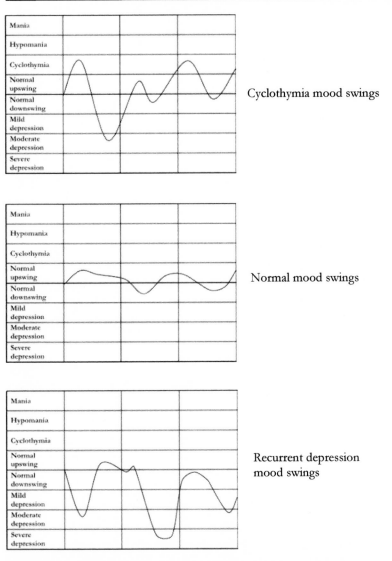

Cyclothymia mood swings

Normal mood swings

Recurrent depression
mood swings

As can be seen from these mood swing graphs, just because an upward mood swing is less severe does not mean that the resulting depression is also less severe. In fact some studies show that bipolar II disorder tends to more disabling as it can be harder to treat and has more residual symptoms than bipolar I disorder in between episodes. Bipolar I disorder is associated with a higher number of co-morbid illnesses such as anxiety disorders, alcohol and substance misuse.

Is lithium better at treating bipolar I, II or cyclothymia?

Most of the studies looking at the effect of drugs on bipolar disorder are done on people with bipolar I disorder. This is because it tends to be easier to define bipolar I. It is clearer when someone has an episode of mania, whereas hypomania and cyclothymia are sometime subject to difficulties in diagnosis.

As a result of this we are often, as doctors, left making decisions about how to treat people with bipolar II (and cyclothymia) based on the research evidence of bipolar I. This may be valid, but in some cases may not be valid. However there is an increasing number of research papers on bipolar II in particular.

Overall treatment of any phase

It is generally accepted that lithium is best overall at treating people with bipolar I disorder and those who have a family history of bipolar I disorder with relatives who have responded well to lithium. This is probably true for treating mania/hypomania, bipolar depression and in maintenance (or mood stabilising) in people with bipolar I.

Lithium is a good drug in treating all phases of the illness in bipolar I and bipolar II disorders. However there is invariably a need to use lithium in combination with other medications.

Lithium appears to be effective but less so in treating those with bipolar II and cyclothymia. This seems to be true in all phases of the illness: going high, becoming depressed and preventing relapses into any mood swing.

Lithium is also an useful mood stabiliser to help stop "switching" with antidepressants. Switching is when antidepressants are given without additional mood stabilisers and cause a hypomanic or manic upswing in mood. The golden rule is that you should not be given antidepressants with bipolar disorder unless you are already on a mood stabiliser. Increasing evidence is also showing that antidepressants may not work and be harmful in many people with bipolar disorder. However there does seem to be a percentage of people with the illness that do respond to antidepressants.

Bipolar Depression

Overall lithium does have antidepressant effects in bipolar disorder overall. However, the size of these treatment effects are smaller than was originally thought, given early research conducted in the 1950s to the 1970s.

There is some evidence that the addition of a second mood stabiliser, in particular sodium valproate, improves lithium's treatment of acute bipolar II depression. There have also been studies looking at the addition of the antiepileptic drug lamotrigine to lithium in treating bipolar depression in both bipolar I and II patients.

Lithium is best at treating depression in bipolar I than II. Furthermore it might be that lithium is less effective in treating depression in cyclothymia than recurrent depression.

Mania / Hypomania / Mood Upswing

Lithium is best at treating mood upswings in bipolar I disorder compared to the upswings in bipolar II disorder and cyclothymia. The evidence for its use in cyclothymia in this way is very limited and likewise poor.

Maintenance Treatment or Mood Stabilisation

The results of medication trials and studies mirror the effectiveness of lithium in other phases of the illness. Lithium is best at maintenance treatment in bipolar I, effective but less so in bipolar II and least effective in cyclothymia. Interestingly, lithium is better at stopping a non-bipolar but recurrent depressive illness than cyclothymia. From this evidence it seems that cyclothymia is clearly the most resistant of these mood disorders to treatment.

Studies have also looked at the blood lithium levels of people with bipolar whilst on long term maintenance treatment. Higher blood levels are more beneficial in mania and hypomania and probably in the prevention thereof. Levels used to effectively treat depression or prevent relapse of depression are lower than in mania.

Chapter Summary

Bipolar I is characterised by mania, bipolar II by hypomania. Cyclothymia is mood swings that are less severe than hypomania. In totality they are called the bipolar spectrum. Each disorder has different outcomes and responses to treatments.

References

Bauer MS et al. What is a 'mood stabilizer'? An evidence-based response. American Journal of Psychiatry 2004, 161, p 3-18.

Calabrese JR et al. Spectrum of activity of lamotrigine in treatment-refractory bipolar disorder. American Journal of Psychiatry 1999, 156, p 1019-23.

Frye MA et al. A placebo-controlled study of lamotrigine and gabapentin monotherapy in refractory mood disorders. Journal of Clinical Psychopharmacology, 2000; 20, p 607-14.

Nemeroff CB et al. Double-blind, placebo-controlled comparison of imipramine and paroxetine in the treatment of bipolar depression. American Journal of Psychiatry. 2001; 158, p 210-16.

Suppes T et al. Lamotrigine for the treatment of bipolar disorder: a clinical case series. Journal of Affective Disorders. 1999; 53, p 95-8.

Thase M. Bipolar depression: Issues in diagnosis and treatment. Harvard Review Psychiatry. 2005; 13, p 257-71.

Young LT et al. Double-blind comparison of addition of a second mood stabilizer versus an antidepressant to an initial mood stabilizer to an initial moos stabilizer for treatment of patients with bipolar depression. American Journal of Psychiatry. 2000; 157, p 124-6.

Chapter Eight

Keeping a Lithium Record and Mood Diary

On the following page you will see a lithium record diary and examples of mood diaries.

It is a good idea to keep a record of the dates and results of your lithium blood tests. This will help you keep up to date with the tests and help you communicate with your doctor on these related issues.

Keeping a diary of your moods over periods of health and mood instability is the best way to understand how your mood changes and how it is affected by changes around you. Presented here are web links to recommended mood diaries, available for free and also iPhone and Android phone apps for you to download that allow you to track and record your moods in a variety of ways.

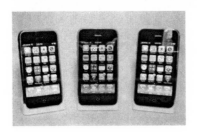

iPhones & Android Phones have apps for all occasions. There are a range of mood monitors

Mood Diaries

Mood diaries can be found at the following websites:

Basic mood diary:
www.psychiatry24x7.com/bgdisplay.jhtml?itemname=mooddiary

Mood diary with instruction including a section for women's issues:
www.bipolar.com.au/common/pdf/mood-diary.pdf

A downloadable mood diary excel version:
www.office.microsoft.com/en-us/templates/mood-diary-TC030007590.aspx

An online mood diary that is also accessible via iPhone app:
www.moodpanda.com/MoodDiary.aspx#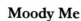

iPhone Mood Diary Apps

Bipolapp
Developed by Cardiff University Bipolar Disorder Research Network, this easy to use app also allows your doctor or nurse to

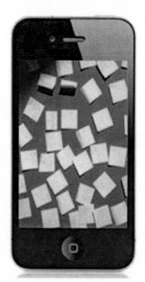

monitor your mood entries remotely and contact you if necessary.

Moody Me
A simple, easy to use but well presented mood diary

NHS Moodometer
A simple app which only allows you to record your mood and plots your current location on a map allowing you to see the mood of others in your area.

Diary Pro lite
Unusual mood diary that automatically records the weather in your area at the time.

Android Mood Diary Apps

Smiley Diary Moods
This is a simple but useful mood app that displays your mood during each day or over days in a variety of graphical forms.

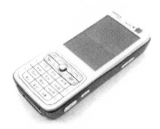

Mood Journal
Basic / Plus / Social-Share
A well designed app that allows you to record not only your mood but also your sleep, medication and weight. It also allows you to remotely share your results with your loved ones or your doctor.

EmoCube Social Diary
This is an easy to use mood tracking app that allows integration with your Facebook and Twitter account.

Lithium Level Record

Date	Dose of lithium	Lithium level	Kidney function (eGFR)	Thyroid function OK?

Date	Dose of lithium	Lithium level	Kidney function (eGFR)	Thyroid function OK?

Date	Dose of lithium	Lithium level	Kidney function (eGFR)	Thyroid function OK?

Date	Dose of lithium	Lithium level	Kidney function (eGFR)	Thyroid function OK?

Date	Dose of lithium	Lithium level	Kidney function (eGFR)	Thyroid function OK?

Glossary of terms

ACE inhibitors
This stands for angiotensin-converting enzyme inhibitors. They are drugs used primarily for high blood pressure and heart failure. Examples include: captopril, enalopril, ramipril, lusinopril and benzapril.

Android phone apps
Software programmes or applications that are designed to run on the Google smart phone operating system. Invariably this means anything that is not an Apple phone.

Akathisia
An unpleasant restlessness that is a frequent side effect of first generation antipsychotics but less commonly associated with second generation antipsychotics.

Amygdala
An area of the brain, and part of the limbic system, that generates emotion based on memory and experience.

Angiotensin II receptor antagonists
These are drugs used in the treatment of high blood pressure, kidney damage due to diabetes and congestive heart failure. Examples include: losartan, telmisartan, irbasartan, azilsartan and valsartan.

Antidepressants
A family of drugs developed and designed to treat non-bipolar depression but also used in the treatment of bipolar depression. There are a number of groups in this family: tricyclics (TCAs), monoamine-oxidase inhibitors (MAOIs), serotonin reuptake inhibitors (SRIs or SSRIs) and serotonin noradrenaline reuptake inhibitors (SNRIs). Examples of these drugs include in the TCA family, lofepramine; in the MAOI family, phenelzine; in the SSRI family, fluoxetine and in the SNRI family, venlafaxine.

Antiepileptic
A drug used in the treatment of epilepsy.

Antimanic
A drug used in the treatment of mania.

Antipsychotic
A drug used to treat psychotic symptoms.

Apoptosis
The natural process of cell death.

App
A software program designed to run on a smart phone.

Autoimmune
A process whereby the immune system turns against the host.

Beta-blocker
A drug that slows the heart rate and reduces blood pressure.
Sometimes use to treat anxiety and panic attacks.

Big Bang
The theory that the beginning of the universe started from nothing
with a large explosion.

Brugada syndrome
A genetic disease that is characterised by abnormal
electrocardiogram (ECG) findings and an increased risk of sudden
cardiac death.

Carbamazepine
An antiepileptic drug that is also used as a mood stabiliser.

Chlorpromazine
A first generation antipsychotic drug.

Clinical research
Research undertaken with the desired outcome to discover something medically meaningful and possibly useful clinically.

Clozapine
An antipsychotic drug which is more effective than any other antipsychotic in the treatment of schizophrenia, but which has dangerous side effects on the bone marrow requiring regular blood tests.

COX2 inhibitors
A form of non-steroidal anti-inflammatory pain killing drug (NSAID) that directly targets COX-2, an enzyme responsible for inflammation and pain. Examples include: celecoxib and rofecoxib.

Delirium
Otherwise known as acute confusional state which is a severe brain syndrome with features of acute onset and fluctuating course, deficits of attention and general disorganization of behaviour.

Depression / Depressive disorder
A state of mind characterised by persistent low mood, low energy and a lack of pleasure in things usually enjoyed. Cognitive features such as concentration, attention and memory problems as well as biological problems such as insomnia are also commonly experienced.

Depressive episodes
Periods of experiencing depression, or depressive disorder.

Depressive relapse
A renewed depressive episode after a period of remission.

Diazepam
A benzodiazepine drug which acts as mild sedative, used principally in anxiety but which can easily lead to addiction.

Diuretics
Drugs which, by acting on the kidney, increase the excretion (removal of) of water.

Divalproex
A form of sodium valproate that is licensed for the treatment of bipolar disorder. Its trade name is 'Depakote'.

DVLA
Driver and Vehicle Licensing Agency, the UK drivers and vehicle licensing agency.

Ebstein's anomaly
A congenital heart abnormality in a newborn child, seen in inceased numbers in children born to mothers on lithium.

ECG
Electrocardiogram, an electrical heart trace. Originally developed on a dog at St Mary's Hospital in London.

EEG
Electroecenphalogram, an electrical brain trace, made by attaching electrodes to the scalp.

Elements
The atoms that combine together to make molecules.

EPSE (extra-pyramidal side effects)
Extra-pyramidal side effects, typically seen with antipsychotics, include Parkinson's-like symptoms and akathisia (see above).

First generation antipsychotics
The first antipsychotic drugs, such as chlorpromazine, haloperidol and sulpride, belong to this family. Their side effects are predominantly effect movement and cause stiffness, difficulty moving and abnormal mouth movements.

First trimester
The first three months of a nine month pregnancy.

Fluid balance
The amount of fluid you consume minus the amount you lose.

Flupenthixol
An antipsychotic drug which is used in higher doses as an antimanic drug and used to be commonly used in small doses as an antidepressant.

Fluphenazine
An antipsychotic drug which can be used as an antimanic.

Follicle
The root of the hair.

Functional brain images
Brain images that show activity, as well as structure, in the brain. Different scanners use different techniques to produce these images. Those more commonly used include fMRI (functional magnetic resonance imaging), PET (positron emission tomography) and SPECT (single-photo emission computed tomography).

Genes
Functional units of DNA that code for proteins.

Genetics
The study of genes.

DNA
Otherwise known as deoxyribonucleic acid. The basic code of genes, consisting of four basic units, which when combined in triplets code for a unit of a protein called an amino acid.

Goitre
Swelling of the thyroid gland.

Hyperthyroidism
Excessive thyroid activity.

Hypervigilance
An enhanced state of sensory sensitivity accompanied by an exaggerated intensity of behaviours whose purpose is to detect threats.

Hypothyroidism
Depleted thyroid activity.

Ibuprofen
A non-steroidal antinflammatory pain killer drug (NSAID).

Idiosyncratic reaction
An unusual individual reaction to a drug.

Iodine
An element that is necessary for the proper functioning of the thyroid gland.

iPhone
The Apple smart phone.

Irritable bowel syndrome (IBS)
A functional bowel condition with no discernable cause characterised by abdominal pain and changing bowel habits.

Lamotrigine
An antiepileptic drug that has been found to be useful as a mood stabiliser, in particular as one that is good at preventing depressive relapses.

Mania
The state of mind of being manic. Characterised by racing thoughts, grandiose delusions, irritability, pressured speech, lack of judgment and excessive spending.

Mefanamic acid
A NSAID that is typically prescribed for period pains.

Messengers
Chemical chain reactions within brain cells that are set off by chemicals and drugs acting at the surface of the cell.

Metronidazole
An antibiotic used for anaerobic infections. Often used in dental infection and severe bowel infections.

Mood stabiliser
A drug that prevents relapse into hypomania, mania or depression. Lithium is the archetypal mood stabiliser.

Myoclonus
A brief, involuntary, twitching of a muscle or muscle group.

National Patient Safety Agency (NPSA)
The NHS body that collects and publishes patient safety and drug information to enable healthcare professionals to improve safe practice.

Neuronal plasticity
The ability of nerve cells to live and re grow and to be resilient to stresses.

Neurotoxicity
Substances that are toxic to and able to cause brain cells to die.

NSAIDS
Pain killers otherwise known as non-steroidal anti-inflammatory drug, such as ibuprofen.

Olanzapine
A second generation antipsychotic drug, originally manufactured by Eli Lilly pharmaceuticals as Zyprexa.

Optic nerve
The cranial nerve that carries information from the retina of the eyes to the brain.

Papules
A papule is a circumscribed, solid elevation of skin with no visible fluid, varying in size from a pinhead to 1 cm.

Parathyroid gland
Small glands attached to the posterior aspect of the thyroid gland, responsible for secreting parathyroid hormone which is involved with the regulation of calcium and other salts.

Parkinson's disease
A degenerative brain condition causing difficulty in walking and other movements. Also associated with depression.

Placebo
A drug containing no active compound. Usually used in drug trials to blindly compare its effectiveness to a new compound.

Prefrontal cortex
The very front of the brain, whose function is primarily executive.

Propranolol
A beta-blocker drug, sometimes used in the treatment of anxiety and panic disorder.

Psoriasis
A skin condition, characterised by silvery scaly plaques, often on the extensor surface of limbs.

Second generation antipsychotics
More current antipsychotics, such as risperidone, olanzapine, quetiapine and aripiprazole. These antipsychotics (on the whole) have less of the movement-related side effects but have other side effects.

QT prolongation
The prolongation of a part of the ECG trace that is often caused by many psychiatric medications. If severe it can cause the heart to go into dangerous rhythms.

Quetiapine
A second generation antipsychotic manufactured by Astra Zeneca under the name of Seroquel.

Risperidone
A second generation antipsychotic manufactured by Janssen Cilag under the name of Risperdal.

Scotoma
A patch of lost vision.

Semisodium valproate (Depakote)
A chemical variation of sodium valproate.

Serotonin
A brain chemical that is associated with mood.

Tetracyclines
An family of antibiotics that have broad activity and a wide range of uses in infections.

Theophylline
A drug used to treat asthma and chronic airways disease.

Thioridazine
A first generation antipsychotic that has now been withdrawn from the market due to safety concerns.

Thyroid gland
The bow tie gland in the neck that is responsible for producing throxine, the hormone that regulates the metabolic rate.

Thyroid stimulating hormone (TSH)
The hormone that is released from the pituitary gland in the brain that tells the thyroid gland to produce more thyroxine.

Thyrotoxicosis
The state of the body when too much thyroxine is produced.

Urea

One of the breakdown products of proteins that is removed by the kidneys.

Valproate

Otherwise known as sodium valproate, an epileptic drug that is also used as a mood stabiliser in bipolar.

Xanthines

Chemicals that are the result of the breakdown of substances from within cells. They are also the chemical building blocks of stimulants, such as caffeine.

Abbreviations

ACE: Angiotensin Converting Enzyme

ADH: Antidiuretic Hormone

BDNF: Brain Derived Neurotrophic Factor

BIH: Benign Intracranial Hypertension

CSF: Cerebrospinal fluid

CANMAT: Canadian Network for Mood and Anxiety Treatments

CJD: Creutzfeld-Jakob Disease

DNA: deoxyribonucleic acid

ECG: Electroconvulsive Therapy

EEG: Electro-encephalogram

eGFR: Estimated Glomerular Filtration Rate

EPSE: Extra Pyramidal Side Effects

IBS: Irritable Bowel Syndrome

IFSBP: International Federation of Societies of Biological Psychiatry

NHS: National Health Service

NMS: neuroleptic malignant syndrome

NPSA: National Patient Safety Agency

NSAIDS: Non-steroidal anti-inflammatory drugs

SILENT: Syndrome of irreversible lithium-induced neurotoxicity

SSRI: Selective Serotonin Reuptake Inhibitor

TSH: Thyroid Stimulating Hormone

UK: United Kingdon

USA: United States of America

YMRS: Young Mania Rating Scale

Index

X